THE JOY OF REFLEXOLOGY

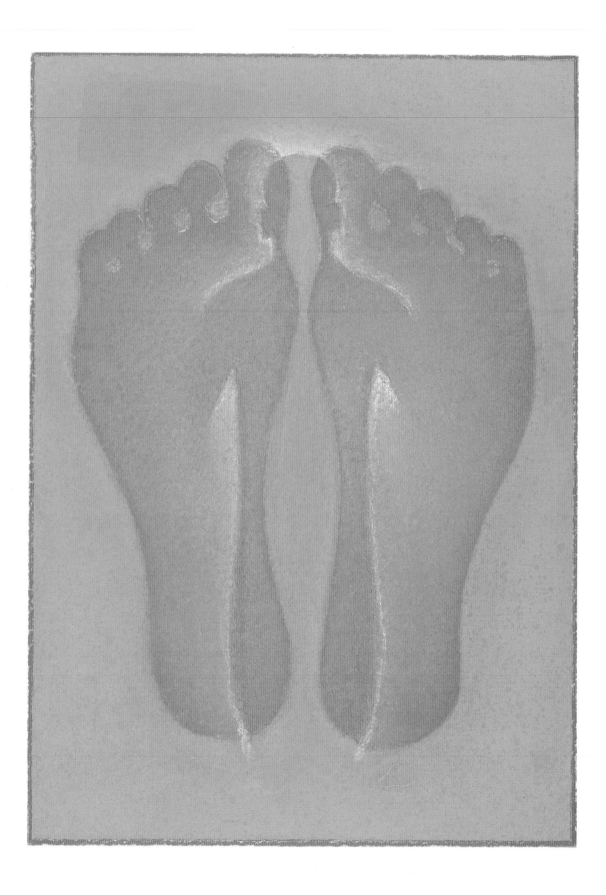

THE JOY OF REFLEXOLOGY

Healing Techniques for the Hands & Feet
to Reduce Stress & Reclaim Health

Ann Gillanders

Little, Brown and Company
Boston New York London

First American Edition

ISBN 0-316-31466-8

Library of Congress Control Number 95-79741

10 9

Printed and bound by MRM Graphics, Singapore

This book is not intended to replace medical care under
the direct supervision of a qualified physician. Before
embarking on any changes in your health regimen, consult
your physician.

Using This Book

Stress is probably one of the most significant factors in our lives. Without it, we would be less likely to find the motivation to strive, to push that little bit harder to achieve our personal goals. Yet stress can also be an extremely negative force in the lives of many people, giving rise to disrupted sleep, personality problems, and a range of organic medical conditions. The first chapter of this book, therefore, emphasizes the link between stress and wellbeing, discusses what stress is, points out the danger signs to watch for, and explains the benefits reflexology can bring.

In order to obtain the maximum benefit from reflexology, you must first understand how the minute reflex points on the feet and, to a lesser extent, the hands relate to and affect the rest of the body. To achieve this, use the body maps of the feet and hands in Chapter Two and the guide to basic reflexology techniques in Chapter Three.

Chapter Four concentrates on all the major systems of the body, such as the respiratory, digestive, reproductive, and circulatory systems. Diagrams show the different components of each system, and text and illustrations explain how these relate to the reflex points on the feet and hands and the specific reflexology techniques you can use to treat them.

Reflexology is a holistic system of treatment. It works best when aimed at the whole person, not focused just on a set of symptoms. Chapter Five sets out, in step-by-step fashion, a complete foot reflexology session, showing you the precise movements and positions of the thumb and fingers on the feet and the order in which the exercises should be carried out to ensure no part of the body is missed. Because foot reflexology requires two people – the giver and receiver – it is not suitable as a self-help therapy. However, you can use hand reflexology on yourself at any time, at home or at work, if you have a complaint or ailment that would benefit from frequent attention. A hand reflexology session is covered in Chapter Six.

The reflexology exercises in Chapter Seven concentrate on treating defined ailments using the reflex points on both the feet and hands. These exercises are not meant to be used in place of a full session, however, merely to supplement it. It is only by carrying out a complete reflexology session will you be alerted to the varying sensitivities of different parts of the feet, which are indicators that perhaps all is not well in specific parts of the body. Finally, a chart of ailments, symptoms, and suggested areas you can treat is given at the back of the book.

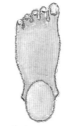

Dorsal view

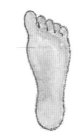

Plantar view

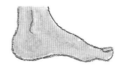

Medial view

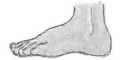

Lateral view

Views of the feet
Throughout this book, references are made to different views or sides of the feet and hands. Although only the feet have been illustrated here, you can easily see how the different views shown also relate to the hands.

Contents

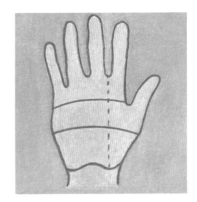

Introduction

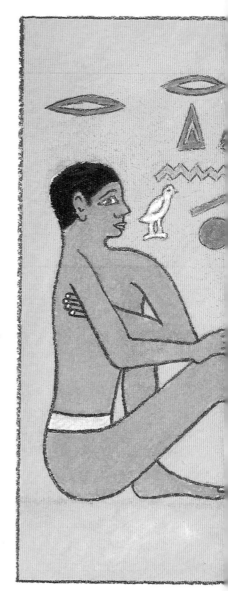

Whether you have a chronic or an acute health problem or you are simply looking for a way to reduce tension and promote wellbeing, reflexology may be the answer to your problem. Although it works on a similar principle to acupuncture, reflexology is entirely non-invasive. Instead of using needles, simple pressure is applied through the fingers to the minute reflex points in and around the feet and hands (*see pp. 24-35*). This, in turn, has a stimulating effect on specific parts of the body.

Reflexology is a completely safe form of therapy, as well as being a very relaxing and pleasant experience. The purpose of a course of treatment is to normalize the body's functioning, to help to break down tension and alleviate stress, and to improve nerve functioning and blood supply throughout the body. The information in this book will allow even a complete novice to relieve many of the troublesome complaints that seem to have become such an unfortunate part of modern life. Reflexology's track record in treating such complaints as painful backs and tension headaches is particularly encouraging. If, for example, you are experiencing an unsettled period in your life, one that is creating tension and anxiety within you, reflexology could give you the support you need in order to cope with your circumstances in a more positive frame of mind.

Reflexology is not effective just with adults, however. You can often soothe a fractious infant simply by applying gentle pressure to the baby's feet – an invaluable technique in the middle of the night, when a few hours of unbroken sleep are desperately needed. As well as babies, young children also seem to have a natural affinity for reflexology, and they are generally very willing to offer up their feet for a soothing treatment. Digestive upsets are another type of problem that can often be easily relieved by reflexology, often far more effectively and safely than any pills or potions.

The principles

The aim of reflexology is to correct the three negative factors involved in the disease process: congestion, inflammation, and tension. Congested conditions are responsible for bringing about growths; inflammatory conditions are those such as colitis, bronchitis, or sinusitis; and tension is responsible for lowering the efficiency of the immune system.

Reflexology sessions are primarily intended to improve the body's circulation and to assist the body in speeding up the

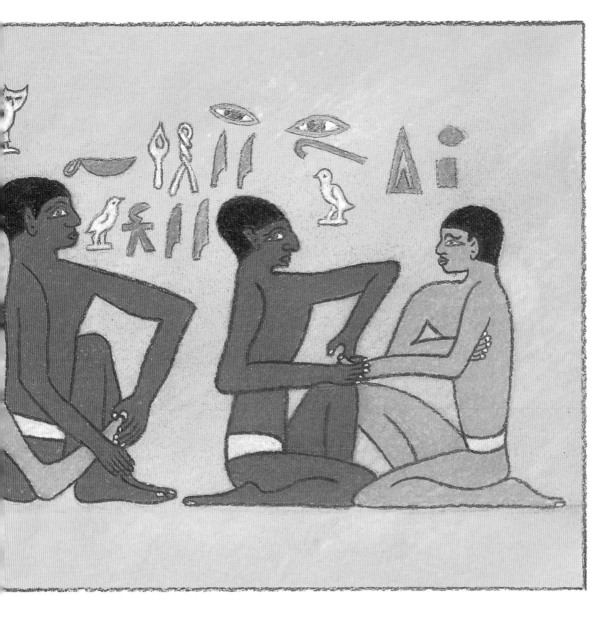

An ancient solution to modern problems
*More than 4000 years ago – as this illustration taken from the
Physician's Tomb at Saqqara, Egypt, shows – the therapeutic benefits of
manipulating specific points on the feet were already known. The
ancient wall painting is full of symbolic meaning. The pyramid shapes
symbolize energy, while the owl represents wisdom and learning, and
the three white birds depict peace, health, and prosperity. The tools that
can be seen in the separate panel are representations of the instruments
used in the surgical procedures of the time.*

elimination of waste products, so that toxins do not have a chance to build up to harmful levels in the liver, kidneys, or bowel. As well, reflexology can help to control the perception of pain by stimulating the release of endorphins – the body's natural painkillers – from the pituitary gland in the brain into the bloodstream. But reflexology works best when it is used to treat the whole body, rather than specific conditions. In this way, it improves all of the body's functions, and this, in turn, encourages the natural healing process to work that more speedily and efficiently.

Hands are meant for healing

The therapeutic benefits of touching are undeniable. It is the most basic form of communication we have; it is an intimate, one-to-one communication that simply has no equal. The tenderness observed between a mother and her newborn child is most often expressed through touch, mainly with the hands. And tension and stresses in your partner, no matter what that person's age, can be sensed through the ultra-sensitive nerve endings of the fingertips and then gently manipulated away.

For the maximum possible benefit, reflexology is always applied to "the very roots of our being" – that is, the feet. This means that two people are required: the practitioner and the receiver. However, as a form of first-aid treatment, you can apply some reflexology techniques to your own hands. Don't then expect this self-help measure to give the same degree of benefit you would get from receiving a full foot reflexology session.

The origins of reflexology

From evidence that we have, reflexology is known to be more than 4000 years old. Paintings discovered in the Physician's Tomb at Saqqara, Egypt, dating back to about 2300 BC, show an actual reflexology treatment in progress (*see pp. 8-9*).

The Chinese are also known to have used reflexology in conjunction with acupuncture. Dr Wang-Wei, a Chinese doctor in the 4th century BC, evidently used to position acupuncture needles in his patients' bodies and then apply very firm pressure with his thumbs to the soles of their feet. This pressure was maintained for several minutes until the desired therapeutic effects were achieved. Dr Wang-Wei maintained that as the pressure was applied and maintained, healing energy was released in the patients' bodies.

The fact that ancient Egypt and China both seem to have shared the same, or similar, knowledge of healing techniques raises the question of whether these two great civilizations had been in contact. Some of the legends associated with the lost island continent of Atlantis tell of great feats of navigation of Atlantean sailors. Perhaps it was they who took information back and forth. This is just a fanciful possibility to highlight that there is no way of tracing the true beginnings of reflexology. But both cultures were great centres of healing in the ancient world and their teachings have spread around the globe.

Reflexology and the West

Reflexology as we now know it in the West has its origins in the study of zone therapy, which utilizes the longitudinal lines of energy running up through the body from the feet to the brain (*see pp. 18-20*). The development of acupuncture was founded on an understanding of these energy zones but, in acupuncture, instead of pressure being applied to specific points, fine needles are inserted under the skin to stimulate the energy pathway and so normalize the workings of the body.

The leading researcher into and popularizer of zone therapy in the West was Dr William Fitzgerald in the early part of the 19th century. Dr Fitzgerald was a graduate of the University of Vermont and, after graduation, worked for two and a half years in Boston City Hospital. Fitzgerald broadened his medical experience oversees, spending time on the staff of the Ear, Nose and Throat Hospital in London and more than two years working in Vienna.

On returning to his native America, Fitzgerald was appointed head of the ear, nose, and throat department of St Francis Hospital in Hartford, Connecticut, and it was here that he brought to the attention of the medical world his research into ancient Chinese healing techniques. His own experiments had led him to discover that by applying pressure to key points on the extremities of the body – principally the feet – he could bring about normal physiological functioning in other parts of the body, no matter how remote these parts might be from the site the pressure was applied to.

A supporter and friend of Fitzgerald's at the time, a Dr Joe Riley, was instrumental in bringing Fitzgerald's discoveries to the notice of a much wider audience. A chance conversation between Riley and Eunice Ingham, a physiotherapist working in a large orthopedic hospital in St Petersburg, Tampa Bay, Florida, was to change the direction of that woman's life. Ingham was immediately fascinated by the potential benefits that seemed to be offered by zone therapy, and introduced reflexology, as we now know it, into her physiotherapy department. To her professional satisfaction, in those patients treated she noted a decrease in their perception of pain, an improvement in their mobility, and, when reflexology was administered directly following surgical procedures, there was a noticeable speeding up of the body's natural healing processes.

So impressed was Eunice Ingham with the results of reflexology that she resigned from her hospital position and started in private practice as a reflexologist in the 1930s. News of her success spread, and people from all over America came for treatment. Ingham went on to write the first book on reflexology and later she was to open the first school specifically to train reflexologists. In all, Eunice Ingham dedicated 40 years of her life to the practice and teaching of reflexology. She died in 1952.

A holistic approach

You would probably not be reading this book if you did not feel that you wanted to help yourself and those around you in some practical way. All of us at one time or another have experienced the distress and upset of seeing friends or loved ones fall sick, and have been moved to help them in some way; to make them feel better or at least more comfortable in themselves.

It is amazing just how dependent we have become on doctors – conventional or complementary practitioners. We put ourselves in their hands and really expect *them* to heal *us*. Some of you may even want to become healers yourselves. Although understandable, these concepts fit poorly into a holistic view of health, however, because they are based on the premise that some people have the power to heal, while others do not.

When I look back at the people I have treated, I know, without a shadow of a doubt, that it is individuals who heal themselves; the practitioner is simply an agent of change. People's health cannot improve until they first have the desire to change and acquire the belief that their health can and will improve.

The majority of people exhaust all forms of conventional medicine – drugs, physiotherapy, surgery, and so on – before, often as a very last resort, they seek out some sort of relief through complementary medicines such as reflexology. It is quite amazing that a patient will happily take prescribed medication for years and years without any particular benefit but then expect reflexology to bring about a completely successful result at the end of two or three sessions. The fact is that it took some time for your health to break down – nobody becomes chronically ill overnight – and therefore it will also take some time for your body to restore itself to equilibrium and balance once more.

Reflexology encourages this healing process to begin. The experience itself does not "heal"; it merely creates the circumstances through which self-healing can occur.

The spiritual awareness that results from reflexology allows you to acquire an insight into the causes of a particular imbalance, and it is this insight that you need to attain before lasting and positive change can take place. The heightened inner awareness developed through reflexology leaves both the practitioner and the receiver with an immense feeling of contentment.

Unfortunately, in most people this fragile awareness is often shielded and submerged by a lifetime of negative psychological self-defence mechanisms that work to the detriment of the individual. By learning to place your trust in the giver of the reflexology treatment, you can take the first step in breaking down these self-defensive barriers.

The communication of touch is an extremely basic instinctive need. Throughout nature we are all well aware of how, for example, young animals not only want but need close contact with their mothers at all times. Adult social animals of all species exhibit this same need for physical closeness and touch, and we are no different.

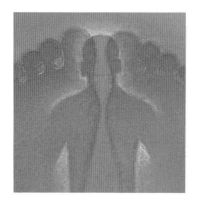

Chapter One
Stress and Wellbeing

Human beings have always been subject to stress, yet we often look back longingly to earlier times when life seemed, from a modern perspective, to have been simpler and freer from pressure and strain. In truth, there has never been an age in human history that was stress free, and each generation has had to deal with an increasingly complex and stressful social environment. Despite the technological advances, especially those of the last few generations that were supposed to usher in a new age of global enlightenment, most of the persistent problems of our planet are even further from solution than they ever were.

Stress factors

What psychological price do we pay in attempting to adjust to the knowledge that war, or its imminence, is with us every day? Do we despair that our scientific knowhow has increased the sophistication of weaponry to the point where the surface of the planet could be rendered sterile for human and most other life for thousands of years into the future? Most of us feel utterly helpless in the face of problems such as these.

Certainly we have hopes that the leaders we elect – and the experts on whom they, in turn, rely – can find the solutions to these types of global problem, but our day-to-day concerns are usually of a more mundane nature (*see opposite*). Our frustrations come about because we generally cannot solve far less earth-shaking problems,

Using the Holmes-Rahe scale

The Social Readjustment Ratings Scale, devised by American doctors T H Holmes and R H Rahe, is a guide to assessing the potentially stress-inducing factors that may be affecting you at any particular point in your life. The 41 positive and negative life events in the chart have each been assigned a value according to the amount of physical and/or mental adjustment required to cope with the event. Those scoring more than 300 units in any one year may have a greatly increased risk of illness. Bringing your score down to 150-299 reduces this risk by 30 per cent, while a score of 150 or fewer carries with it only a slight risk of illness. Since individual responses to particular situations vary so greatly, you should regard your score as only a crude indicator of the way you are reacting to levels of stress.

The Holmes-Rahe scale	
Life event	**Life change units**
Death of a spouse	100
Divorce	73
Marital separation	65
Imprisonment	63
Death of a close family member	63
Personal injury or illness	53
Marriage	50
Dismissal from work	47
Marital reconciliation	45
Retirement	45
Change in health of a family member	44
Pregnancy	40
Sexual difficulties	39
Gain of new family member	39
Business readjustment	39
Change in financial state	38
Change in frequency of arguments with spouse	35
Major mortgage	32
Foreclosure of mortgage or loan	30
Change in responsibilities at work	29
Son or daughter leaving home	29
Trouble with in-laws	29
Outstanding personal achievement	28
Spouse begins or stops work	26
Begin or end school	26
Change in living conditions	25
Revision of personal habits	24
Trouble with boss	23
Change in working hours or conditions	20
Change in residence	20
Change in schools	20
Change in recreation	19
Change in church activities	19
Change in social activities	18
Minor mortgage or loan	17
Change in sleeping habits	16
Change in number of family reunions	15
Change in eating habits	15
Vacation	13
Christmas	12
Minor violation of the law	11

such as getting to work on time through traffic-choked city streets. Indeed, the everyday demands of living make it more and more difficult to escape the increasingly adverse psychological effects that seem to be built into our existence. Whatever it may be – daily commuting, the rising cost of living, incessant noise, air pollution, emotional disharmony at home, unemployment, or random violence – most of us find it difficult to reach a satisfactory inner equilibrium and, as a result, we are prone to some degree of negative stress.

As well as having a psychological component, stress can also affect you physiologically, undermining your immune system and general health and leading to such problems as hypertension, heart disease, and strokes. Many orthodox doctors today accept that about 75 per cent of all illnesses they treat stem from stress-related conditions. Good doctors are also becoming increasingly sensitive to the types of patient who may be particularly prone to such diseases as arteriosclerosis, high blood pressure, gall stones, and arthritis due to stress.

Positive aspects of stress

Stress is not all negative. It can be a very positive feature in our lives, since we all need to be under a certain degree of stress to be able to perform at our best in many types of demanding situation. If, for example, you limp through life like an overstretched spring it is unlikely you will feel the motivation to set and achieve goals.

Positive stress also plays a part in our ability to relax and enjoy ourselves. The stressful, exuberant emotion experienced when you are watching your favourite soccer team score that winning goal, for example, is a positive factor, as is the type of stress reaction that motivates you to climb a rock face or strain to beat your personal best time in a running race. It is only when you are constantly stressed and on "red alert", even when you try to "turn off" at night and sleep, that stress becomes harmful.

Stress is part of our evolutionary heritage. The hunter-gatherer societies that still survive today give us some insight into the role stress has to play in terms of basic survival. When a successful hunt can mean the difference between having sufficient to eat and going hungry, the physiological changes your body undergoes due to stress are extraordinary. When stalking your prey, with every nerve in your body quivering, the pupils of your eyes dilate to improve your long-distance vision. Your adrenal glands start to produce extra adrenaline, which in turn raises your pulse rate and increases your heart beat. Fat and sugar are extracted from the liver to give you more energy, blood pressure rises, and your heart rate increases even more. By now you are aware that your rate of breathing has increased and even your hearing is more acute. With the extra adrenaline you are able to run faster because your body is receiving a higher level of oxygenated blood. Eventually you make your kill. The energy expended in killing your prey and then dragging it back home burns up your remaining energy reserve.

This scenario illustrates how the body should work in any stress-inducing situation: excess adrenaline is produced to help you achieve your goal, and this is followed by physical exercise to use up the excesses the body has produced. However, today most of us are subject to the physiological changes due to stress without the exercise needed to redress the imbalances created.

Stress management

In order to achieve a state of wellbeing we need to pay attention to our bodies' basic needs – sleep, relaxation, good nutrition, physical exercise, and a change of attitude to the factors in our lives that are creating negative stress reactions. Ask yourself whether you allow time to enjoy leisure activities, some part of the week that is reserved just for you, to relax, to swim, to read, to practise a hobby?

A part of a stress-management routine could include a relaxing reflexology session – a monthly treatment would be perfect for most people to help preserve good health. It is puzzling why we most often turn to complementary or orthodox treatment only when our bodies are already sick, when a regular maintenance programme could prevent problems occurring and help promote wellbeing.

Diet is another vitally important aspect of stress management – you will get more out of your body in terms of performance if you are careful about what you put into it in the first place. If you are stressed or run down, it is essential to avoid stimulating foods – those containing caffeine, for example, or food colourings, additives, and preservatives – since these may have a profound, anxiety-producing effect on many people.

If you smile into a mirror it can only smile back at you; frown into one and the reflection is returned to you. What we give out of ourselves we will ultimately receive back. It is impossible to give out love and positive feelings and receive back hatred and disharmony.

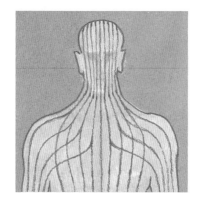

Chapter Two

The Principles of Reflexology

Reflexology is based on the presence of ten energy zones within the body. These zones are longitudinal, ascending from the base of the body – the feet – right through to the top of the head. This energy division was discovered in the late 19th century by an American, Dr William Fitzgerald, an ears, nose, and throat specialist. While working in hospitals in Paris, Vienna, and London, Fitzgerald discovered that he could relieve pain in one part of a patient's body by applying pressure to another part (*see pp. 11-12*). He refined his technique, learning that if he applied pressure to the fingers by using an elastic band on the middle segment of each finger and a small metal clamp on each tip, he could create local anaesthetic effects on the arm, side of the neck, eye, ear, and face.

You need to bear in mind that at the time Dr Fitzgerald was practising, in the 1880s, anaesthetics were very crude. Chloroform masks were used, and more patients died as a result of the anaesthetic than of the surgery.

Mapping the zones
The body is divided into ten energy zones, five on each side of the spine. The zones run from the toes and then up through the head, with zone 1 starting at the big toe. The hands also form part of the zone map, with zone 1 starting at the thumb.

The ten energy zones
What do we do instinctively when suffering from a headache, say, or an upset stomach? We usually place our hand on the aching area to obtain some relief. So as a very basic instinct, we all use pressure to relieve pain symptoms.

The ten zones are arranged in five pairs, numbered 1-5, on each side of the body. Zone 1 runs through the thumbs on both sides and then through the inside central line of the body, the front inside

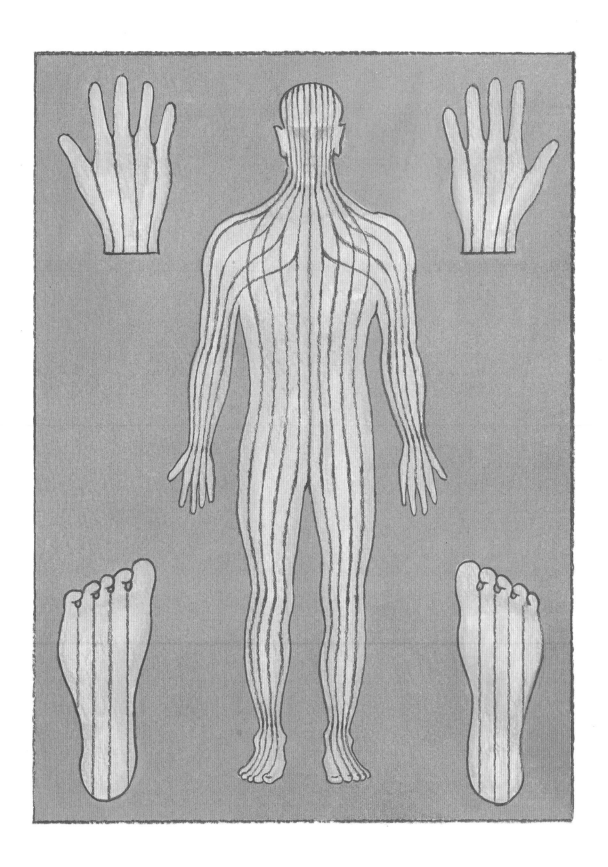

legs, inside arms, inside body, and through the area of the spinal column. Any impairment of energy flow here may affect any organ or function falling within this zone. Because so many vital parts of the body are found here – nose, mouth, throat, spinal column, and sex organs – zone 1 is usually by far the most sensitive in people's feet. By simply working on the spinal reflexes in the feet it is possible to relieve a host of unpleasant physical manifestations, since nerves stemming from the area of the spine stimulate the functioning of the entire human body.

Zone 2 takes in the area of the body from the index finger to the second toe, and so we can proceed through the body, dividing it up into ten slices.

This method of dividing the body up into energy channels, or meridians, is similar to the principle underlying both acupressure and acupuncture. When reflexology is taught, however, the meridians themselves are not emphasized and nor are the meridian points identified or numbered. Instead, the emphasis is placed on the body map showing that each area and organ of the body is mirrored on the soles and toes of the feet and the palms and fingers of the hand. The other important difference between reflexology and acupressure or other meridian-based healing therapies is in the thumb and finger techniques used to relax the reflex points in the feet and hands (*see pp.36-7*).

Electrical mapping

Hiroshi Motoyama, a Japanese healer and physician, has studied the zones and acupressure meridians and also electrically mapped the meridian endings, which he calls *seiketsu*, in the fingers and toes. To achieve his results, Motoyama has devised machinery to detect energy blockages by measuring the changes in the electrical impulses in the meridian endings, and he is thus able to diagnose disease before its physical manifestation. This is similar to the way a reflexology practitioner is able to free the tense, granular-like deposits in the meridian endings of the hands and feet that correspond to the different functions and organs of the body.

Motoyama's work verifies what healers have known for centuries: when a meridian point is blocked, the energy flow is decreased or overloaded and congestion develops at that spot. At some later time, this congestion may manifest itself physically as a *dis-ease* of that body part or organ. If, on the other hand, the blockage is removed by a course of reflexology, and the correct balance and normal functioning of the body is restored, the self-healing process can begin and the symptoms and pain will disappear.

Many, if not all, of the complementary healing skills are based on the simple principle of releasing blocked energy flows to bring about the healing process. Perhaps when more research has been carried out, the medical establishments will discover what complementary practitioners have always known.

Guidelines to the hands and feet

In order to understand reflexology it is essential to study the guidelines on the feet and hands identified in the illustrations below. These lines simply divide the feet and hands into broad sections and, by so doing, we are indirectly dividing up the body into areas. Bear in mind that in reflexology the feet, in particular, absolutely mirror the body (*see pp. 22-3*).

The diaphragm line on the feet is just below the metatarsal bones. It is easy to find because the skin colour above the line is darker than the skin colour below. On the hands, the diaphragm line is about 1in (2.5cm) down from the join of the index finger to the hand.

On the feet, the waist line is in the middle of the foot. You can identify it by running your index finger along the outside of the foot

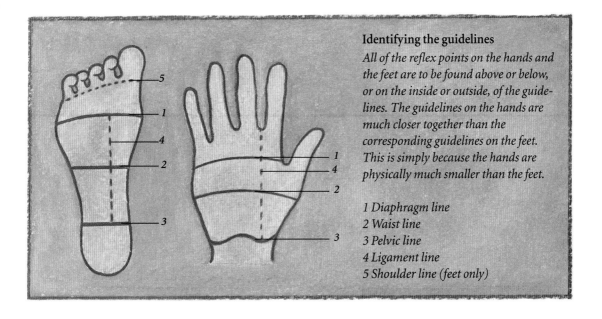

Identifying the guidelines
All of the reflex points on the hands and the feet are to be found above or below, or on the inside or outside, of the guidelines. The guidelines on the hands are much closer together than the corresponding guidelines on the feet. This is simply because the hands are physically much smaller than the feet.

1 Diaphragm line
2 Waist line
3 Pelvic line
4 Ligament line
5 Shoulder line (feet only)

until you reach a small bony protrusion – the metatarsal notch. From this notch, draw your line across the foot. This indicates the area of the waist of the person you are about to work on. If you are a long-waisted person, then the notch will be lower on the foot; if you are high-waisted, the notch will be higher on your foot. On the hands, look for the waist line where the thumb joins the hand.

The pelvic line on the feet is located at the base of the heel: you can find it by placing your index fingers on the inside and outside ankle bones and drawing a line between them. On the hands, the pelvic bone commences at the soft, fleshy part of the pad of the thumb, about 1in (2.5cm) down from the wrist.

To find the ligament line on the feet, pull the big toe back and just between the groove of the first and second toes you will feel a tight, elastic-like vertical ligament. On the hands, the ligament line will be found starting between the second and third fingers.

The shoulder line, which is referred to as a secondary line, is only found on the feet, and is located just below the base of the toes.

The feet: a mirror of the body

If you study the foot chart shown on the right, it quickly becomes obvious how the feet precisely mirror the body. This is even more evident when you have had a chance to familiarize yourself with the guidelines diagram of the feet (*see p. 21*).

Looking at the illustration opposite, you can see that the right foot governs the right-hand side of the body, and the left foot the left-hand side. When you bring the two feet together, you have a complete outline of the human body, with the big toe representing the head and the lateral sides of the feet reflecting the outside of the body – the shoulders, knees, and hips, for example.

Certain external conditions of the feet can be highly significant. A bunion, for example, may often reflect a neck condition, and a sensitivity in the neck reflexes points on, say, the right foot would be significant to a bunion on the same side. A build-up of hard skin on the lateral side of the foot, in line with the shoulder reflex points, often identifies a shoulder condition.

It is difficult to conduct a thorough reflexology treatment session if you have to miss out certain areas because of corns, callouses, and areas of hard skin, so do encourage the people you intend to treat to take good care of their feet. It has been said that the pains in your feet are reflected in your face, and this is very true.

Feet and body
If you look at the two feet (opposite), you can see that they are an exact representation of the human body. The feet really do reflect body type. Those with large, wide shoulders have wide feet from the toe joint to the outside edge. Tall, slim people tend to have long, slim feet with long toes. Note, too, that the curves of the feet look just like the curve of the spine.

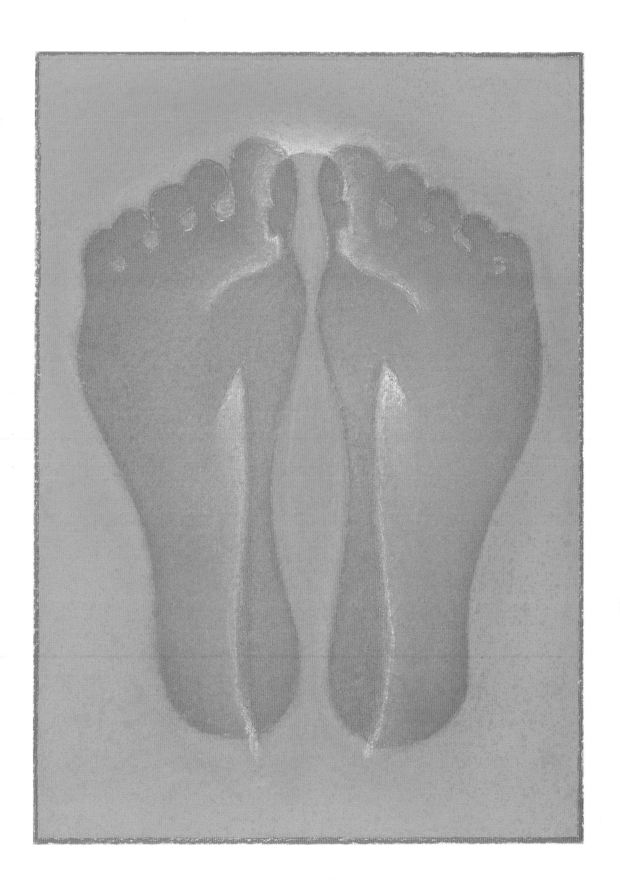

The Feet – Plantar View

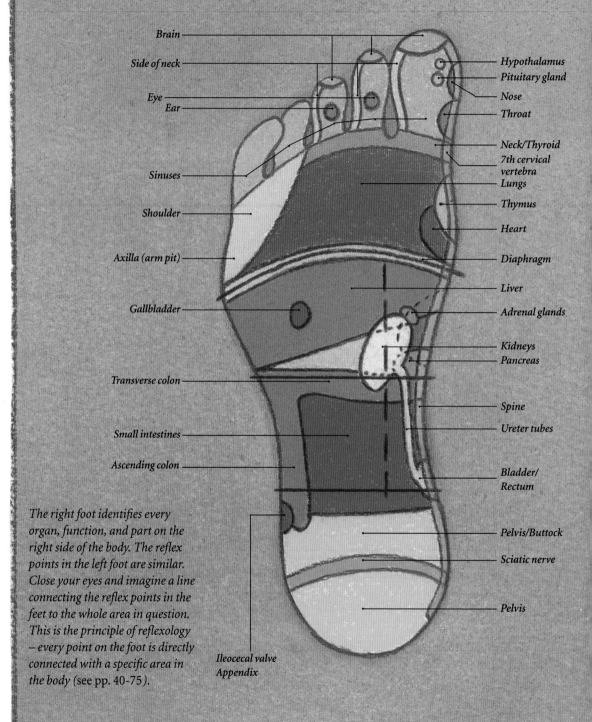

Brain
Side of neck
Eye
Ear
Sinuses
Shoulder
Axilla (arm pit)
Gallbladder
Transverse colon
Small intestines
Ascending colon

Hypothalamus
Pituitary gland
Nose
Throat
Neck/Thyroid
7th cervical vertebra
Lungs
Thymus
Heart
Diaphragm
Liver
Adrenal glands
Kidneys
Pancreas
Spine
Ureter tubes
Bladder/Rectum
Pelvis/Buttock
Sciatic nerve
Pelvis

Ileocecal valve
Appendix

The right foot identifies every organ, function, and part on the right side of the body. The reflex points in the left foot are similar. Close your eyes and imagine a line connecting the reflex points in the feet to the whole area in question. This is the principle of reflexology – every point on the foot is directly connected with a specific area in the body (see pp. 40-75).

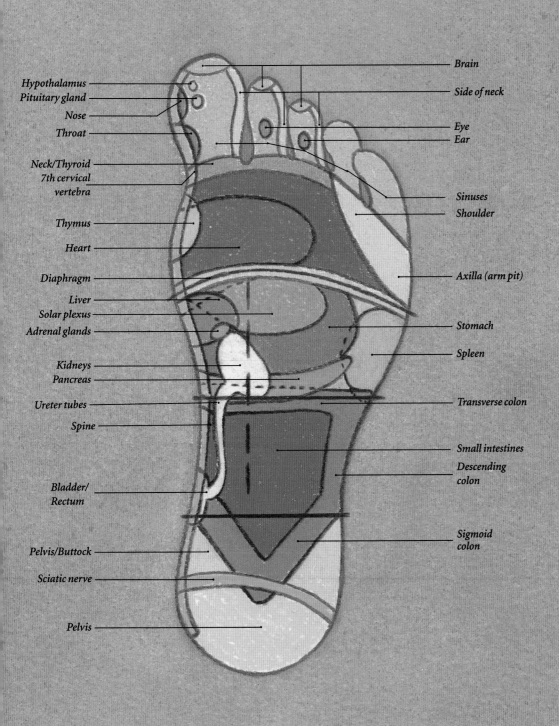

Hypothalamus
Pituitary gland
Nose
Throat
Neck/Thyroid
7th cervical vertebra
Thymus
Heart
Diaphragm
Liver
Solar plexus
Adrenal glands
Kidneys
Pancreas
Ureter tubes
Spine
Bladder/Rectum
Pelvis/Buttock
Sciatic nerve
Pelvis

Brain
Side of neck
Eye
Ear
Sinuses
Shoulder
Axilla (arm pit)
Stomach
Spleen
Transverse colon
Small intestines
Descending colon
Sigmoid colon

The Feet – Dorsal View

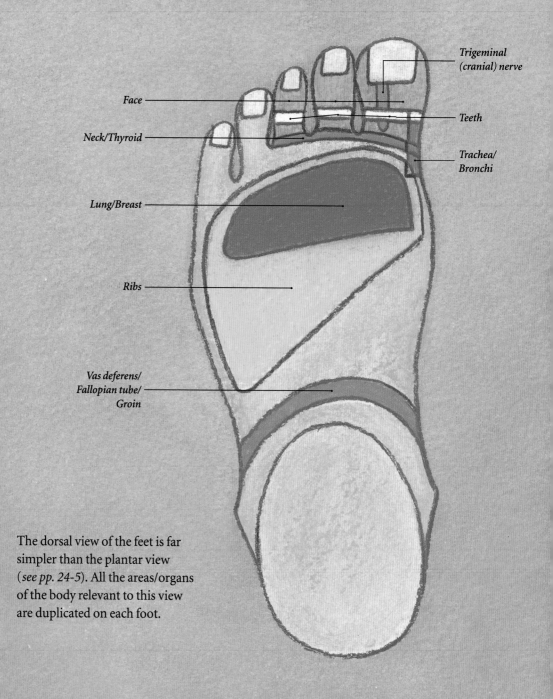

Trigeminal (cranial) nerve

Face

Teeth

Neck/Thyroid

Trachea/ Bronchi

Lung/Breast

Ribs

Vas deferens/ Fallopian tube/ Groin

The dorsal view of the feet is far simpler than the plantar view (*see pp. 24-5*). All the areas/organs of the body relevant to this view are duplicated on each foot.

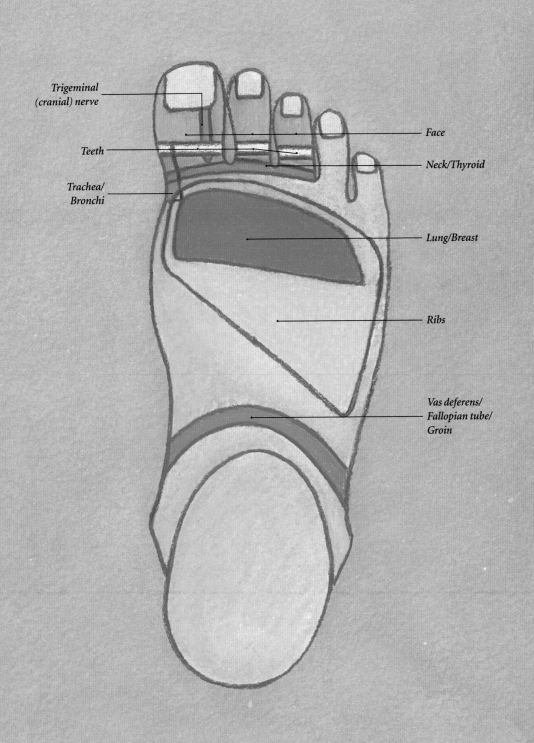

Trigeminal (cranial) nerve

Teeth

Trachea/ Bronchi

Face

Neck/Thyroid

Lung/Breast

Ribs

Vas deferens/ Fallopian tube/ Groin

The Feet – Lateral View

The lateral view of the foot contains only a very few reflex points. However, the reflex point for the muscular area of the upper arm is to be found here, in particular the biceps, which often become strained through too much lifting. The bony structure of the hip joint and the large, winged formation of the pelvis can be found at the very base of the heel, and the link to the ovary in the female and the testis in the male.

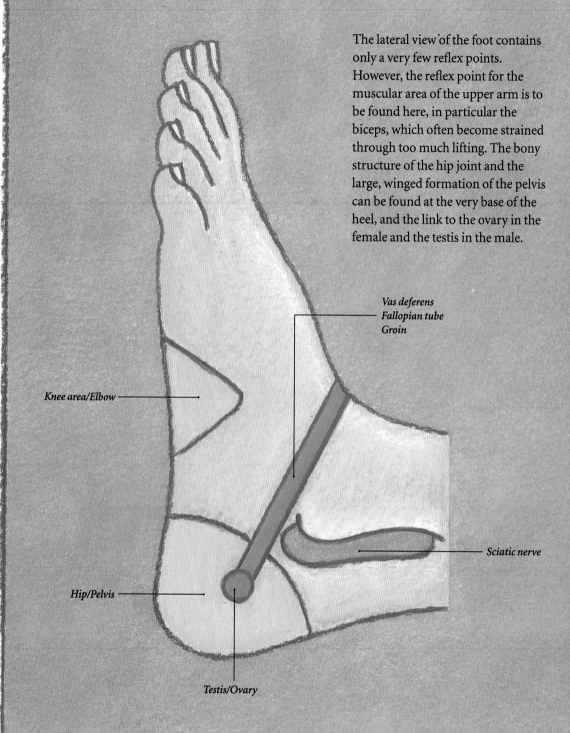

Knee area/Elbow

Vas deferens
Fallopian tube
Groin

Sciatic nerve

Hip/Pelvis

Testis/Ovary

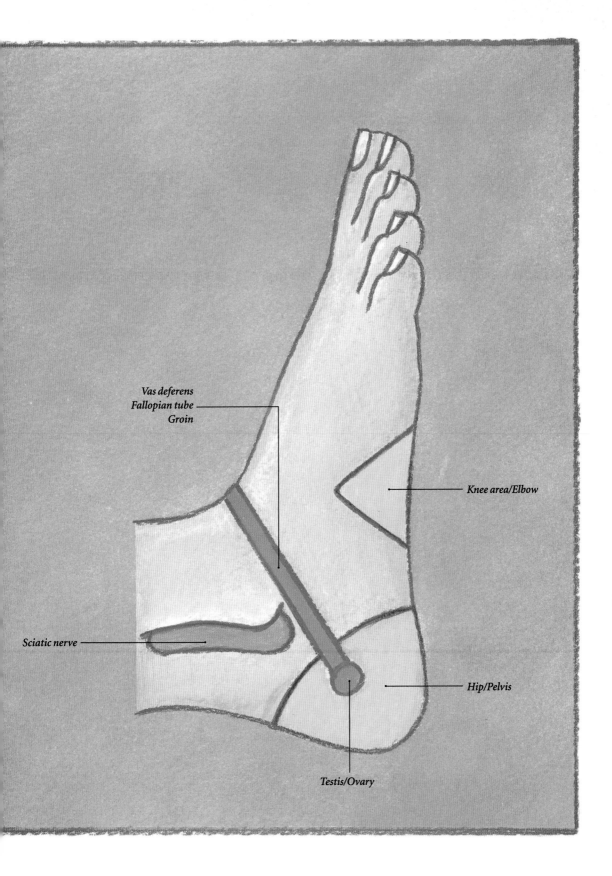

Vas deferens
Fallopian tube
Groin

Knee area/Elbow

Sciatic nerve

Hip/Pelvis

Testis/Ovary

The Feet – Medial View

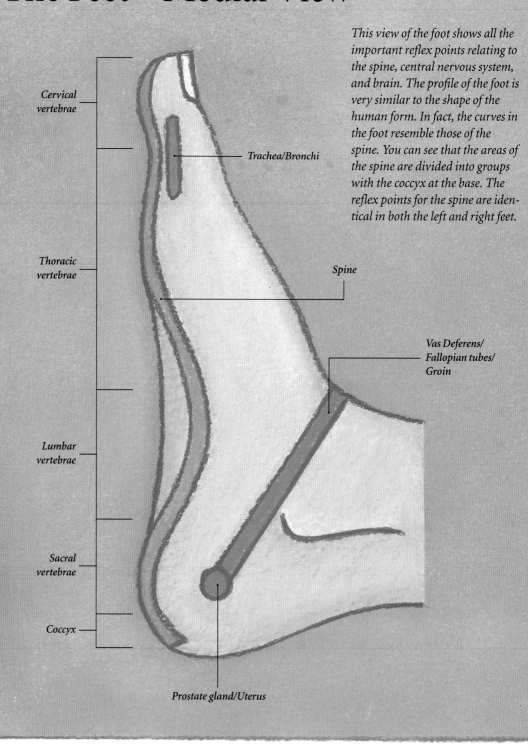

This view of the foot shows all the important reflex points relating to the spine, central nervous system, and brain. The profile of the foot is very similar to the shape of the human form. In fact, the curves in the foot resemble those of the spine. You can see that the areas of the spine are divided into groups with the coccyx at the base. The reflex points for the spine are identical in both the left and right feet.

Cervical vertebrae

Trachea/Bronchi

Thoracic vertebrae

Spine

Vas Deferens/ Fallopian tubes/ Groin

Lumbar vertebrae

Sacral vertebrae

Coccyx

Prostate gland/Uterus

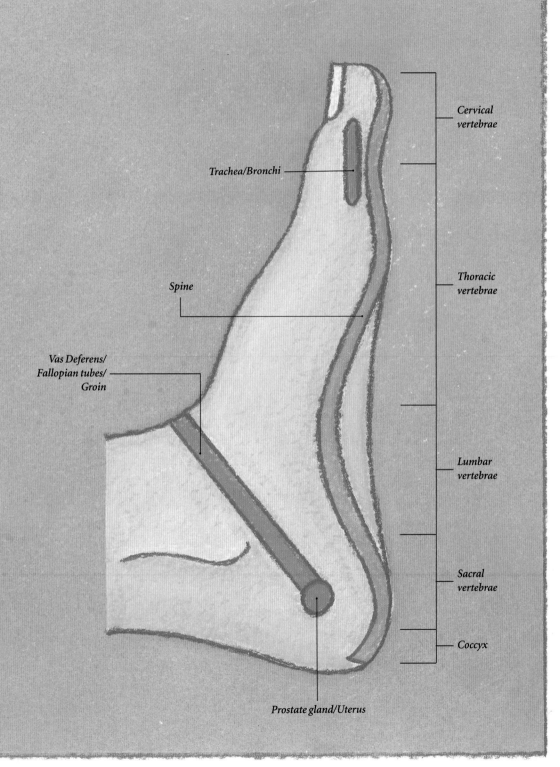

Cervical
vertebrae

Trachea/Bronchi

Thoracic
vertebrae

Spine

Vas Deferens/
Fallopian tubes/
Groin

Lumbar
vertebrae

Sacral
vertebrae

Coccyx

Prostate gland/Uterus

The Hands – Plantar View

The reflex points for the head, eye, ear, sinus, and lung areas are identical on the palms of both the right and left hands. The changes occur in the arrangement of the reflex points to the organs on the left and right sides of the body.

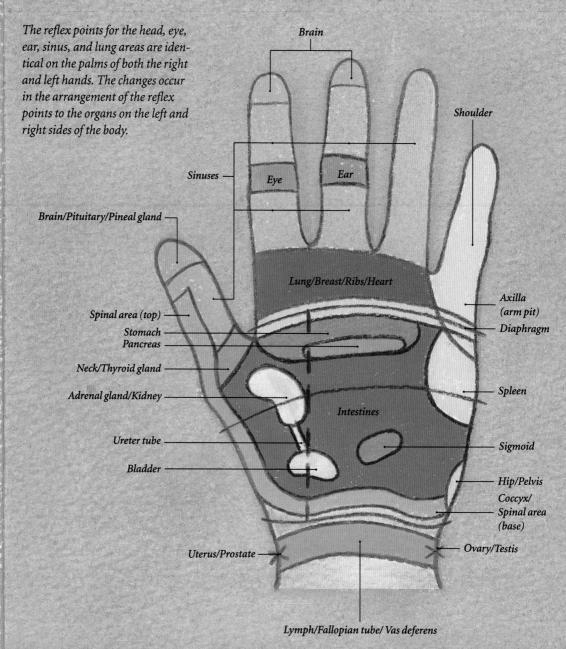

Brain

Shoulder

Sinuses

Eye

Ear

Brain/Pituitary/Pineal gland

Lung/Breast/Ribs/Heart

Axilla (arm pit)

Spinal area (top)

Diaphragm

Stomach

Pancreas

Neck/Thyroid gland

Adrenal gland/Kidney

Spleen

Intestines

Ureter tube

Sigmoid

Bladder

Hip/Pelvis

Coccyx/ Spinal area (base)

Uterus/Prostate

Ovary/Testis

Lymph/Fallopian tube/ Vas deferens

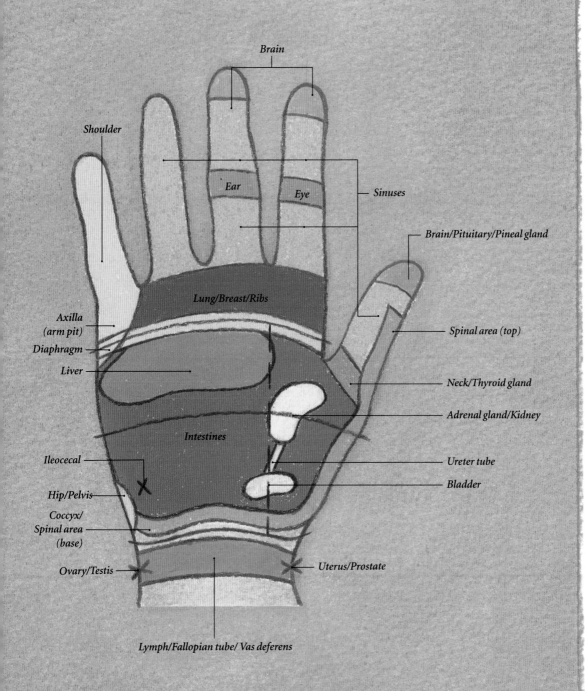

Brain

Shoulder

Ear

Eye

Sinuses

Brain/Pituitary/Pineal gland

Lung/Breast/Ribs

Axilla
(arm pit)

Diaphragm

Liver

Spinal area (top)

Neck/Thyroid gland

Adrenal gland/Kidney

Intestines

Ileocecal

Ureter tube

Bladder

Hip/Pelvis

Coccyx/
Spinal area
(base)

Ovary/Testis

Uterus/Prostate

Lymph/Fallopian tube/ Vas deferens

The Hands – Dorsal View

If you visualize the continuation of the guidelines in the plantar view (see pp. 32-3) around the dorsal view of the hands, the identifying features become the same. The profile of the hands is so narrow that it is not necessary to show a medial or a lateral view.

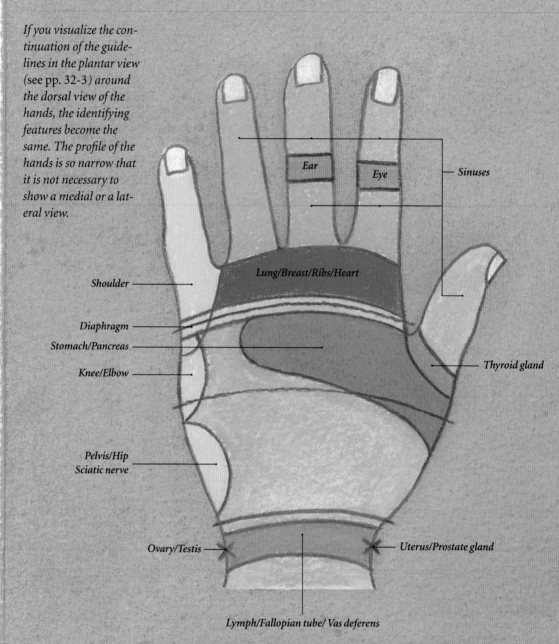

Ear

Eye

Sinuses

Lung/Breast/Ribs/Heart

Shoulder

Diaphragm

Stomach/Pancreas

Knee/Elbow

Thyroid gland

Pelvis/Hip
Sciatic nerve

Ovary/Testis

Uterus/Prostate gland

Lymph/Fallopian tube/ Vas deferens

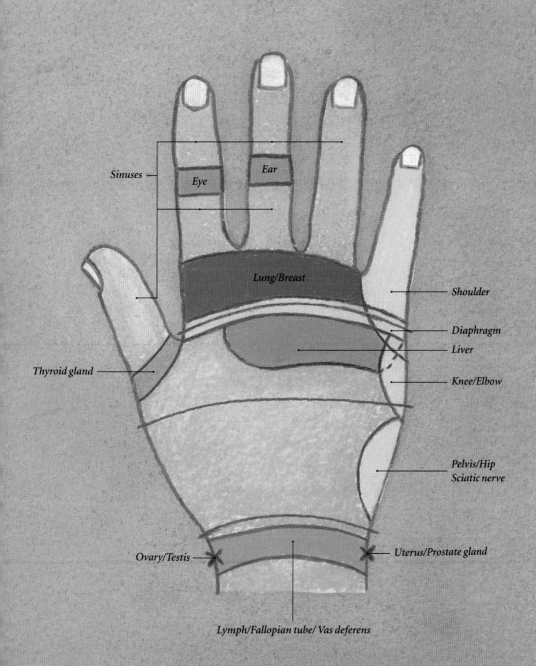

Sinuses

Eye

Ear

Lung/Breast

Shoulder

Diaphragm

Liver

Knee/Elbow

Thyroid gland

Pelvis/Hip
Sciatic nerve

Ovary/Testis

Uterus/Prostate gland

Lymph/Fallopian tube/ Vas deferens

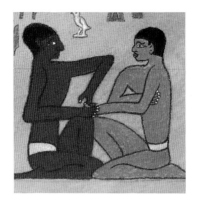

Chapter Three

Basic Techniques

Using your thumb and index finger correctly while giving a reflexology treatment is vital if you are to achieve the best possible results. The reflex points are minute and there are thousands of them distributed on the feet and hands. So that no points are missed, each movement of your thumb or index finger must be precise and disciplined. Imagine an old-fashioned type of pin cushion displaying an array of pins positioned with just tiny gaps between each – your thumb or finger must press down on the head of each pin in turn.

The direction of movement of the thumb or finger is always forward and never backward; and avoid circular movements and any type of sliding technique. Another important point to bear in mind is that you should never use the very tip of your thumb or finger when giving a reflexology treatment. Instead, use the flat, pad part of the digit – otherwise your nail may dig into the skin of the receiver's foot, or the skin of your own hand if you are using reflexology as a self-help technique (*see pp. 88-97*), which can be uncomfortable or even painful. Long nails are definitely out for reflexologists!

One of the commonest questions asked by people learning basic reflexology techniques is : "How much pressure should I apply?" This must largely be intuitive. If you were working on your own hands, for example, it would be difficult to imagine creating too much pressure, since the hands can tolerate a lot of force. But as a guideline when working on somebody's feet, which are more sensitive than the hands, you should never use so much pressure that the receiver flinches or tries to withdraw his or her feet.

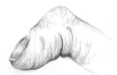

Too arched

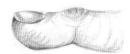

Too flat

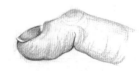

Correct

Finger techniques

The thumb or finger movement is similar to the movement of a caterpillar, with the digit moving only about ¹⁄₁₆in (1.5mm) at a time. The movement is always forward, never circular or sliding.

It takes time to develop the necessary strength and control in your thumb and index finger required to give a reflexology treatment. As you develop the essential techniques, you will gradually learn to achieve a smooth, consistent pressure, one that makes the treatment an enjoyable experience for the receiver.

Keep uppermost in your mind some basic facts: the reflex points are tiny and so your thumb and finger movements must be small and disciplined; movements are always forward, never backward; use the flat pads of your fingers, not the tips, to prevent your finger or thumb nails digging in; pressure must be firm yet not so hard to produce discomfort or pain.

You may be tempted to apply oil or cream to a receiver's hands or feet before a treatment. Don't! Slippery skin makes good contact with the reflex points impossible.

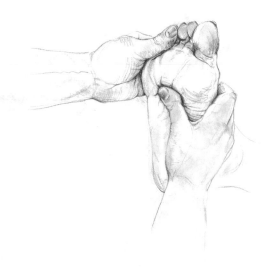

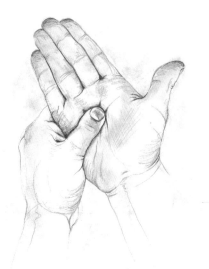

Basic working procedures
When working on the reflex points of somebody's foot or your own hand, bear in mind that each individual point is tiny. You must work slowly and methodically in order to achieve a disciplined and thorough coverage of a particular area. Once you have learned this technique, you have mastered the true art of reflexology.

Working the hands and feet

Since working the hands is a self-help technique, you will have only one hand free at a time. This makes treatment more limited than when working on somebody else's feet. Use a creeping movement over the palm, working in a criss-cross fashion. Work up the fingers with your thumb, then turn your hand over and work down from the bases of the fingers toward the wrist, using your index finger.

If you are working on the receiver's right foot, support it in your left hand and use your right thumb to give the treatment, starting at the medial edge (*see p. 5*). As long as you match right thumb to right foot or left thumb to left foot you are commencing correctly.

Supporting your hand

To work on your own hands, place the hand to be treated on a small cushion on your lap and support it with your other hand. If you contact a sore reflex point, work on and over that particular area again. Spend about 10 minutes working on each hand.

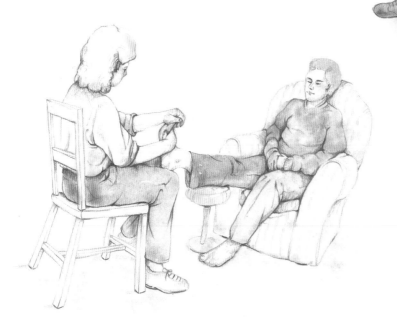

Supporting the feet

Seat the receiver in a comfortable reclining chair or garden lounger. To work on the sole of the foot and any area above the waist line (see p. 21), support the top of the foot. To work on areas below the waist line, support the heel.

Hooking out and rotating

Apart from the creeping, forward motion of the thumb or index finger, there are two other techniques – "hooking out" and "rotating" – but use these only when extra stimulation is needed. There are three areas where these techniques should be applied. First, you can use rotation on the kidney reflex point (*see pp. 24-35*), which can become inflamed due to an excessive intake of caffeine, food colourings, or additives. Second, rotation can also be applied to eye-ear reflex points. Finally, hooking out can be used on the ileocecal valve reflex point to help ease all manner of intestinal complaints.

► **Hooking out**

The ileocecal valve reflex point is on the right foot or hand only, located on the lateral edge near the pelvic line. Press down on this line, applying pressure with your left thumb. Then, draw your thumb back so that it describes the shape of a fish hook.

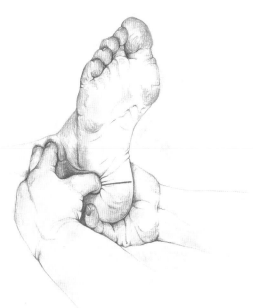

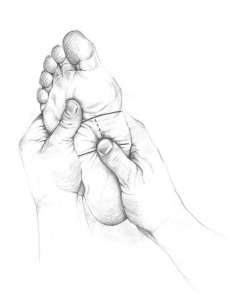

◄ **Rotating**

To use the rotating technique, place the flat of your thumb on the relevant reflex point and rotate the foot or hand around the thumb. Leave the thumb pressure on the point for several seconds to achieve maximum benefit.

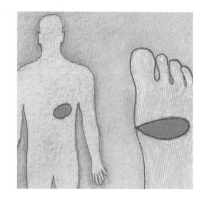

Chapter Four

Understanding the Body Systems

This chapter will give you a good insight into how the body works, where all the major organs and parts of the body are to be found, and how these organic structures relate to the work of reflexology. As we saw earlier, the feet perfectly mirror the human body (*see pp. 22-3*). As you become accustomed to the notion that the feet are channels of healing for all the body systems, and not just the two structures on which we stand, and often treat with utter disrespect, reflexology will start to have a proper context.

Bedside manner

Doctors of old had little to offer their patients over and above the types of herbal remedies that had been used by healers for countless generations. It was only comparatively recently that the first manufactured drugs became available – mild painkilling tablets, bottles of cough medicine, laxatives, and various "rub-in" remedies for painful joints or muscular strains.

Bear in mind that until recently manual labour for most people was the norm – in the home and at work – and an extremely effective and much-used concoction for the resulting sprains and strains was known as "horse oil" – a mixture of wintergreen, camphor, juniper, and liquid paraffin. Its name derives from the fact that it was originally used to treat horses that had gone lame. However limited their practical skills, doctors would normally remain with their patients during a "healing crisis", particularly in the cases of pneumonia, bronchitis, or rheumatic fever. As a result, doctors

Animal instincts

Our early ancestors discovered some of the principles of healing by observing how animals cured themselves when ill. Wild animals first seek out solitude, somewhere they can completely relax. A feverish animal quickly hunts up an airy, shady place near water, there remaining quiet, eating nothing at all, and drinking frequently until it has recovered. A rheumatic animal finds a spot in direct sunlight and lies there as the pain is slowly baked out of its system.

tended to be judged more on their bedside manner – the peace of mind and comfort that they could bring to their patients – than on their ability to effect an actual cure.

This type of one-to-one communication and care has largely been lost today, submerged in the need to treat more and more patients. And with an increasingly aging population, doctors have less and less time to spare to treat their patients, let alone to sit with them through a healing crisis. This is where the true benefits of reflexology can arise, for people of all ages. The provision of just an hour of comforting, relaxing treatment on a weekly basis, an hour of completely undisturbed time, is a precious commodity in the hustle and bustle of modern life.

Learning through illness

Disease is an integral part of the human condition. There is no possible way that we can eliminate it from our lives. Humankind has evolved through health and sickness, and we learn from both.

We have learned to view sickness as bad, and so we attack it by any means at our disposal, even through the administration of powerful drugs that we only partly understand. Any hint of discomfort is responded to by an over-the-counter cure-all or a prescription. Often, the drugs we take do nothing to cure the problem, but only mask its symptoms. The body has its own mechanisms for coping with physical imbalances and drugs often interfere with these processes.

A holistic approach to healing views the body as a dynamic energy system that is in a constant state of change. Humans are more than their bodies. Each is a complex balance of mental, physical, and spiritual aspects that are integrated into and directly affected by environmental and social factors. The causes of illness are far deeper rooted than merely their external symptoms. But we live in an age of scientific specialization, and so each part of the body is viewed and treated as being separate from the rest.

In orthodox medicine, drugs, physiotherapy, and, as a last resort, surgery are some of the treatments used to alleviate pain and discomfort. The aim of reflexology is to achieve the same results, at least with many common complaints, by relaxing the patient and relieving nervous tension (*see pp. 14-17*). Reflexology is increasingly losing its status as a fringe therapy, to the extent that, over the past few years, several teaching hospitals have taken reflexologists into their physical medicine departments.

The Digestive System

Reflexology is proving to be particularly successful in treating many of the common, yet debilitating, conditions relating to the digestive system. Because of its function, the digestive tract is highly reactive to the types of food and drinks we ingest, as well as being very prone to upset in stress-sensitive individuals.

The digestive system comprises the mouth, liver, gallbladder, stomach, pancreas, ileocecal valve, ascending colon, transverse colon, descending colon, small intestines, and sigmoid colon.

The stomach lies tucked up in the abdomen at the level of the lower rib line. The stomach acts as a reservoir for food. When empty, it resembles a deflated balloon; when full, however, the 35 million glands lining its walls secrete up to 80fl oz (3.5l) of gastric juice (mainly hydrochloric acid) per day in order to prepare food for entry into the duodenum – the first part of the small intestine.

The liver is the largest organ in the body and, in an adult, weighs between 2.6 and 4lb (1.2 and 1.8kg). It lies in the right side of the upper abdomen, where it is protected by the ribs. One of the vital substances the liver produces is bile, which is stored in the gall-bladder. Bile salts break down fat and, thus, assist in the absorption of dietary fat and fat-soluble vitamins.

The pancreas is about 6in (15cm) long and lies behind the stomach and in front of the spine. The pancreas performs two important functions: it produces blood sugar, which is fuel for the cells; and it produces insulin, which regulates the level of blood sugar in the body.

You can think of the intestines as being an elaborate food-processing plant in the shape of a long, flexible tube. The function of the intestines is to make the food passed from the stomach acceptable to the body. The first part of the intestinal tract is the small intestine, made up of the duodenum, about 10in (25cm) long, the jejunum, about 8ft (2.4m) long, and the ileum, about 12ft (3.6m) long. Next is the large intestine, which, although wider than the small intestine, is considerably shorter – only about 5ft (1.5m) long in total. The large intestine is divided into the ascending, transverse, descending, and sigmoid colons.

Any material that the intestines cannot process, such as dead bacteria, lubricating mucus, and rough, fibrous material that cannot be absorbed, is passed through the anus and out of the body.

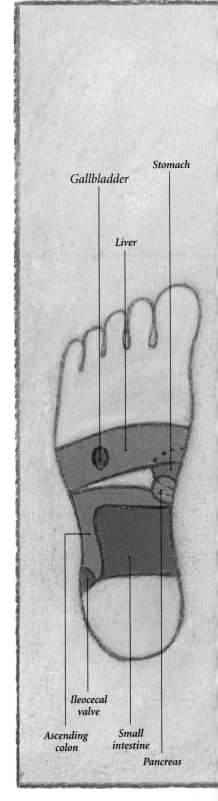

Stomach

Gallbladder

Liver

Ileocecal valve

Ascending colon

Small intestine

Pancreas

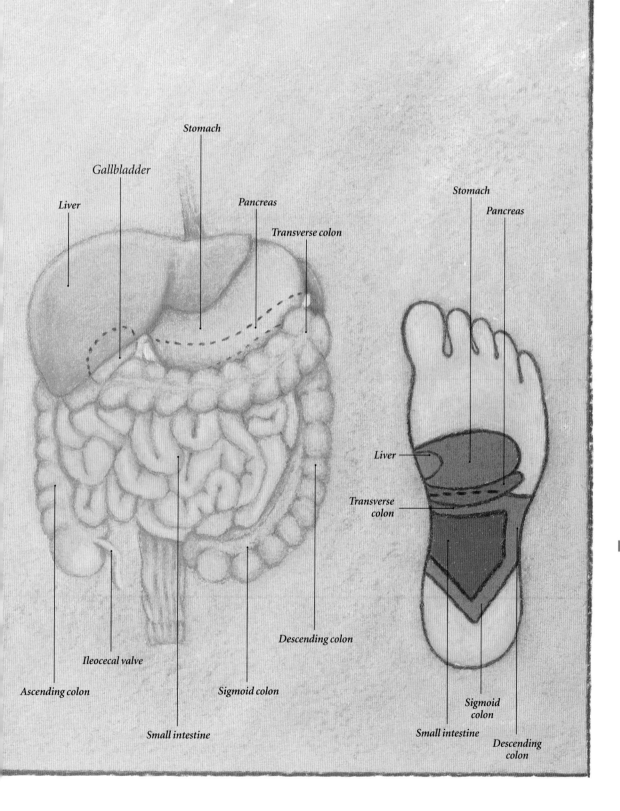

Stomach

Gallbladder

Liver

Pancreas

Transverse colon

Stomach

Pancreas

Liver

Transverse colon

Ascending colon

Ileocecal valve

Small intestine

Sigmoid colon

Descending colon

Small intestine

Sigmoid colon

Descending colon

The digestive system and reflexology

The digestive system is complex. Its activities can be summarized as ingestion, chewing, and swallowing, which means taking food into the mouth and mechanically breaking it down. Next, food is converted into soluble compounds in the stomach and nutrients are extracted in the intestines. Any substances that cannot be digested are excreted by the bowels. Many of these processes can be upset by stress and tension, and so reflexology has had particular success in relieving such problems as irritable bowel syndrome, diverticulitis (an inflammation of the colon), constipation, and general gastric conditions of the stomach.

► **Working the liver and gallbladder**

To treat these areas, support the right foot with your left hand and use your right thumb to work from the medial to the lateral side of the foot between the waist and diaphragm lines. Change your supporting hand and now use your left thumb to work back from from the lateral to the medial side of the foot.

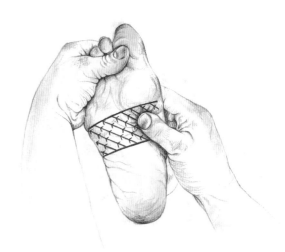

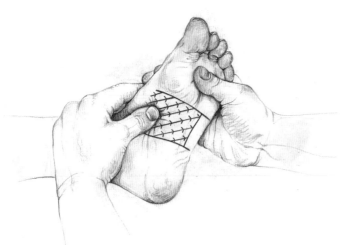

◄ **Working the stomach and pancreas**

Support the left foot with your right hand, use your left thumb and work on the reflex points for the stomach and pancreas from the medial to the lateral side. Change your supporting hand, and then use your right thumb to work on the reflex points from the lateral to the medial side.

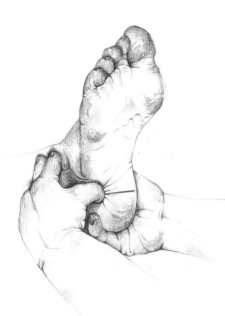

◄ **Working the ileocecal valve**

To treat this area, support the right foot at the base of the heel with your right hand. Next, place your left thumb on the heel line of the foot and use the hooking-out technique (see p. 39) on the relevant reflex point.

► **Working the ascending, transverse, and small intestine**

Support the right foot with your left hand and use your right thumb to work the entire area from the waist line to the very base of the heel. Work from the medial to the lateral side. Then, change your supporting hand and use your left thumb to work the area from the lateral to the medial side.

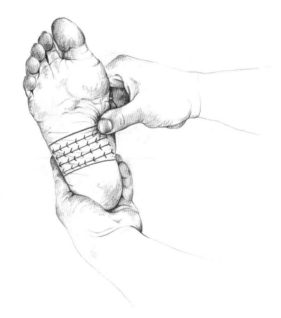

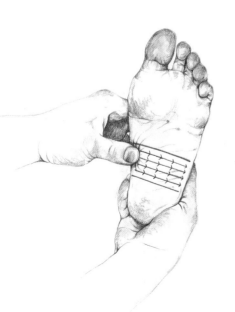

◄ **Working the transverse, descending, and sigmoid colon and small intestine**

Supporting the base of the left foot with your right hand, use your left thumb to work out the entire area from the medial to the lateral side. Change your supporting hand and use your right thumb to work the area again from the lateral to the medial side.

The Reproductive System

Reflexology has proved to be very successful in regulating hormonal functioning related to the male and female reproductive systems. It has, for example, a very direct effect on normalizing the uterus and ovaries during menstruation (*see p. 48*) and, in the male, on maintaining the healthy functioning of the prostate and testes.

Due to the radically different organs making up the reproductive systems of the male and female, the following information is broken down into two parts. Many of the reflex points for comparable or equivalent organs, however, are common to both sexes.

The male anatomy

The reproductive system of the male comprises two testes, the vasa efferentia, which joins each testis to the vas deferens, and this, in turn, connects with the urethra in the centre of the prostate gland. The seminal vesicle acts as a storage organ for the mature sperm.

The prostate gland lies around the first part of the urethra at the base of the bladder, and its secretions help to maintain sperm activity. The penis, as well as being the male organ of reproduction, also has the function of excreting urine from the bladder out of the body.

The testes have two functions: the production of about 50 million sperm cells each day and the production of the hormone testosterone. This hormone is responsible for the development of the male's secondary sexual characteristics. These include pubic and facial hair growth, aggressiveness, muscle bulk, and a deep voice.

The female anatomy

As well as producing a ripe ovum, or egg, once a month, the female reproductive system has to provide nutrition and protection for a fertilized ovum until it develops into a mature fetus at the end of the term of pregnancy. At the top of the vagina, situated behind the bladder and in front of the rectum, lies the uterus, or womb. The uterus is held in place by a series of muscles and ligaments attached to both the pelvic floor and the side of the pelvis. This small, pear shaped organ, which is the nursery of new life, is protected by a thick wall of interwoven muscle fibres.

The monthly cycle of changes the uterus undergoes is amazing, and each change is under the control of hormones produced in the ovaries (*see p. 48*). The uterus has three openings: two fallopian tubes (one from each ovary) enter the upper part of the uterus, while the cervix, or birth canal, is located at the base

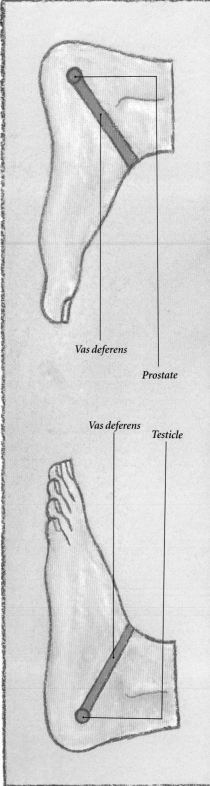

Vas deferens

Prostate

Vas deferens

Testicle

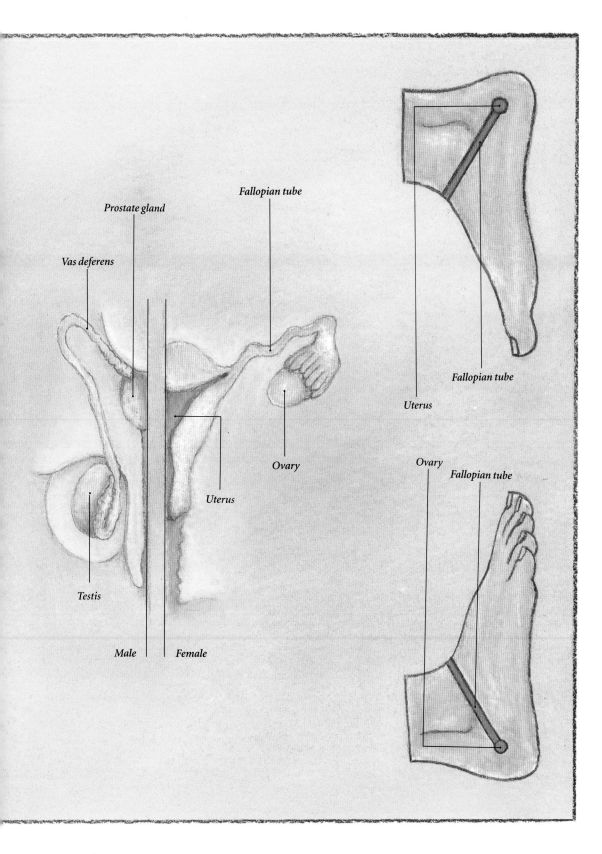

Vas deferens

Prostate gland

Fallopian tube

Fallopian tube

Uterus

Ovary

Uterus

Ovary

Fallopian tube

Testis

Male

Female

The ovum, which first matures and ripens in the ovary, is swept down the fallopian tube and into the uterus by a combination of ciliated epithelium – literally, the rhythmic beating of the minute threads that project from the surface of the cells lining the tube – and wave-like peristaltic muscular contraction.

Estrogen, which is sometimes referred to as the "youth hormone", is produced in the ovaries. During a woman's reproductive years, the presence of estrogen throughout the body helps the skin, hair, internal organs – particularly the heart – and the major arteries to remain healthy.

Unlike the male urinary system (*see p. 46*), that of the female is entirely separate from the reproductive system. The bladder empties into the urethra, which opens in front of the vagina.

The ovaries and the menstrual cycle

The ovaries have two principal functions: the production and ripening of ova (eggs) and the secretion of the hormones estrogen and progesterone. At the age of puberty, usually between the ages of 11 and 14, the sex glands become functional and menstruation begins. Secondary sexual characteristics also become apparent, such as enlarged breasts, the growth of pubic hair, and a redistribution of fat to the buttocks and shoulders. These changes are the result of the effect on the ovaries of an increasing pituitary secretion of follicle stimulation hormones (FSH) and luteinizing hormones (LH).

Each of a woman's ovaries contains anywhere between 50 and 250,000 ova. However, only approximately 500 of these are ever likely to mature and ripen during the woman's reproductive life. During each menstrual cycle of about 28 days, ovulation occurs and one of the ovaries releases an ovum – a single cell almost invisible to the naked eye – into its connecting fallopian tube. If the ovum is fertilized during its five-day journey down the fallopian tube, the ovum implants itself in the wall of the uterus. If it is not fertilized, however, the ovum – along with the blood-engorged lining of the uterus – is expelled into the vagina and then out of the body.

Each stage of the menstrual cycle is controlled by a complex series of hormonal secretions. Infrequent, or even absent, periods can be the result of hormonal imbalances brought about by emotional upsets and stress (*see pp. 14-17*).

Reflexology as an aid to fertility

Because the correct functioning of the reproductive systems of both the male and female is so susceptible to stress and tension, reflexology can be of great benefit. In women, menstruation can cease completely if stress levels become too high, and men in similar situations may find it impossible to maintain an erection. Many couples who had experienced difficulties in conceiving a child have reported successful conception after extensive courses of reflexology.

► **Working the ovaries/testes**

Support the right foot with your right hand and, using your left index finger, work the area indicated in a straight line 2 or 3 times. Supporting the left foot with your left hand, use your right index finger to work the area as before, 2 or 3 times.

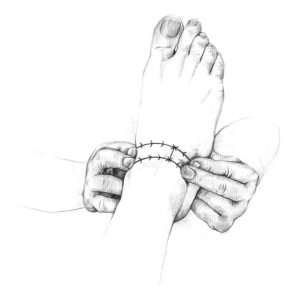

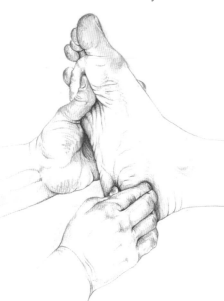

◄ **Working the uterus/prostate**

Support the right foot with your left hand and, using your right index finger, work the area in a straight line. Repeat this process 2 or 3 times. Support the left foot with your right hand and use your left index finger to work the area as before. Again, repeat this 2 or 3 times.

► **Working the fallopian tubes/vas deferens**

Supporting the plantar side of the right foot , pressing in for support with both thumbs, work around the front of the foot with your index and third fingers together 2 or 3 times. Repeat this sequence on the left foot.

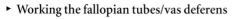

The Respiratory System

The respiratory system is concerned with breathing and supplies all the cells of the body with the oxygen they need for processing food to produce energy. The key organs in this process are the lungs – two spongy bags that occupy most of the chest cavity.

Air breathed in through the nose or mouth is first warmed and moistened as it passes through the nasal passages and pharynx, which is part of the alimentary canal situated between the mouth and the esophagus. Air continues down the trachea, or windpipe, except when this breathing tube is momentarily shut off by a flap of skin, known as the epiglottis, when you swallow. Next, the trachea branches into two bronchi, which take the air into the lungs.

Inside the lungs, each bronchus divides into small tubes called bronchioles, which, in turn, culminate in what are known as alveolar sacs. Looked at more closely, each alveolar sac is composed of tiny chambers called alveoli, whose walls support the network of extremely fine blood vessels called capillaries. It is through the walls of these capillaries that the exchange of gases actually occurs, with oxygen passing into the bloodstream and carbon dioxide and other waste products passing out into the alveolar sacs.

The mechanics of breathing

Working in unison, a large sheet of diaphragm muscle, which is located in the area of the chest below the lungs, and intercostal muscles, designed to move the ribs up and down, squeeze and expand the lungs somewhat like an old-fashioned pair of bellows.

As you breathe in, the ribs move up and out and the diaphragm moves down to elongate the chest cavity. This expands the chest and draws air into the lungs through the air tube connecting the nose and mouth with the lungs.

When you breathe out the opposite occurs: the ribs move down and in and the diaphragm moves up. This has the effect of contracting the chest cavity, thus forcing the air, which now contains carbon dioxide and other waste products, up and out of the body through the nose and mouth.

Vocalization

Another important aspect of the respiratory system involves our ability to make sounds, or to vocalize, which is due to special structures located in the body's airway. Exhaled air from the lungs flows through the larynx, which is also knows as the voice box. The larynx

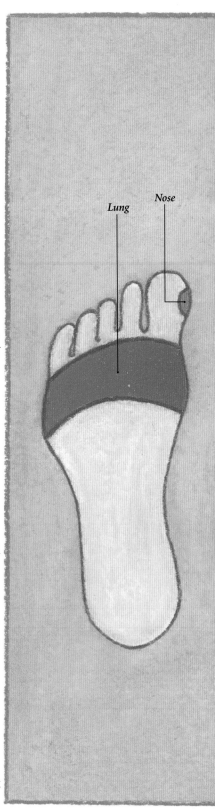

Lung *Nose*

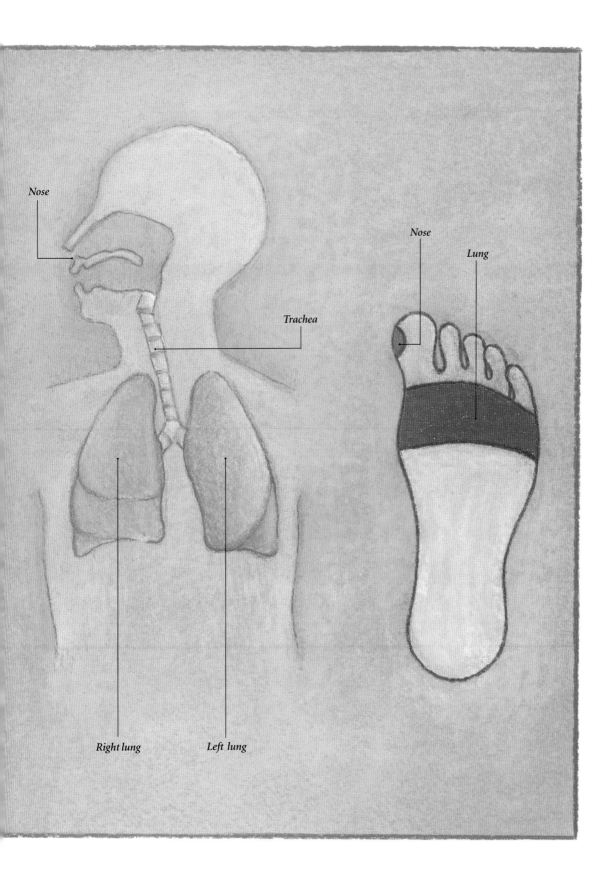

Nose

Trachea

Right lung

Left lung

Nose

Lung

is a broad part of the upper windpipe protected by tough thyroid cartilage that forms the visible bulge in the throat known as the Adam's apple.

Two bands of tissue, the vocal cords, form a V-shaped opening across the larynx. As we speak, these cords tighten and so restrict the opening. Exhaled air then causes the cords to vibrate and so sound is produced. The length of the cords determines the pitch of the sound, in exactly the same way as a guitar or violin string changes pitch depending on its length and tautness – the longer and tauter the cord, the higher its pitch. It is not only the length of the vocal cords that determines the characteristics of the sounds we make, however. Sounds also vary due to the different positions of our tongue, lips, and teeth. The nasal cavity, too, changes the quality of the sounds we make by giving resonance to the voice.

Respiration and digestion

Lifestyle, including dietary factors and the generally poor state of the environment we live in, has a dramatic impact on the respiratory system. Reflexology has had encouraging success with upper respiratory tract infections, bronchitis, emphysema, and asthma (*see opposite*).

Although it may be difficult to accept initially, some problems of the respiratory system are often connected with digestion, and in order to obtain relief from them you may need to work the reflex points connected with the digestive system (*see pp. 42-5*).

There is evidence that by introducing infants to too wide a range of foods at too early an age, some of them may acquire respiratory problems while still very young. The fashion for feeding infants as young as 6 weeks of age on high-protein cereals and dairy products, for example, can stress their immature digestive systems and lead to episodes of infection in both the upper and lower respiratory tracts. These infections can start as inner-ear conditions in the first few months of life, followed by constant catarrh. If this persists, the child may then start to exhibit symptoms of what is sometimes described as wheezy bronchitis.

It is important to remove all dairy-based products and wheat-based cereals from the diet of affected children in order to give their digestive systems a chance to recover. This change in diet, linked with frequent reflexology sessions, often brings about exceptionally good results.

Asthma

Asthma is an increasingly troublesome condition and may even be life threatening in some instances. But by working on lung function and helping, in particular, to relieve the anxiety and strain associated with this extremely distressing ailment, many people have found a remarkable improvement in their overall health. Children, especially, seem to respond well to reflexology treatments, with attacks becoming either less frequent or less severe. In some cases, they have even stopped altogether.

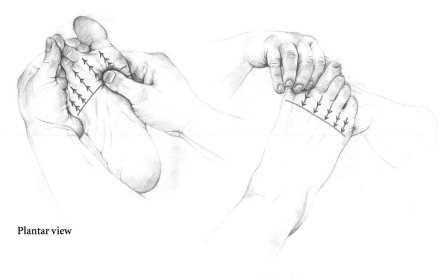

Plantar view

Dorsal view

Working the lung/breast

Starting with the plantar view, support the right foot with your left hand, and work up the area from the very base of the diaphragm line to where the toes join the foot. With the dorsal view, make a fist with your left hand and press it into the plantar side side of the right foot. Use your right index finger to work down the grooves in the foots. Repeat these steps on the left foot.

The Circulatory System

Angina and other coronary conditions respond well to reflexology. The main benefits are in helping muscular function, improving blood supply and nerve functioning, and in helping the general health of an individual by reducing stress levels. The heart is associated with the left-hand side of the body and so you will find its reflex points predominantly on the left foot.

Structure of the heart

The heart, which is central to the body's circulatory system, is a muscular pumping organ. Beating continuously more than 100,000 times a day, it is responsible for circulating blood to every cell in the body. The heart is divided into two halves, each with a thin-walled atrium and a thicker-walled pumping centre, or ventricle. The chambers on each side of the heart are separated by a valve that controls the blood flow between them. Deoxygenated blood enters the heart via the right atrium. It is then forced through the valve into the right ventricle. From there, the blood is pumped to the lungs via the pulmonary artery. Oxygenated blood from the lungs travels back to the heart through the pulmonary veins and enters the left atrium and passes into the left ventricle, from where it is pumped through the aorta to be circulated around the body.

The beating of the heart is controlled by the autonomic nervous system. In this way, your heart continues to beat when you are asleep, for example, or the number of heart beats increases during strenuous exercise to satisfy your extra need for oxygenated blood.

The circulation of blood

Arteries are the largest blood vessels and carry oxygenated blood from the heart to the body and cells. The smallest blood vessels are the capillaries, and it is through the walls of the capillaries that blood passes to nourish the surrounding tissue. From the capillaries, blood flows into the veins and then back to the heart. Contractions in muscles surrounding the veins keep the blood on the move, and special valves ensure that it cannot flow in the wrong direction.

Each time your heart beats it sends a pulse through your arteries. For most healthy adults, the pulse rate is approximately 70 beats per minute, but it is more rapid in children and slower in elderly people.

Blood pressure is the pressure your blood exerts on the walls of your arteries. It varies, depending on how fast the heart beats and on the condition of the arteries themselves.

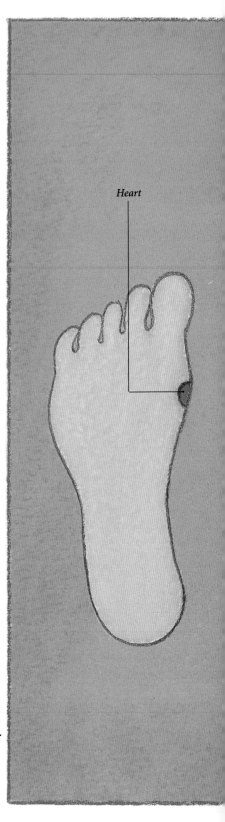

Heart

Working the heart reflex points

Since the heart and lungs function together like a reliable team, you will already have treated the heart area when you worked on the respiratory system (see pp. 52-3). Don't overwork this area, however. Proceed in one direction only, support the top of the left foot with your right hand, and use your left thumb to work in horizontal lines.

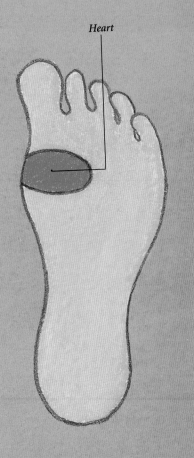

Heart

Heart

The Lymphatic System

Since the lymphatic system is distributed throughout the body, there is no need to isolate specific reflex points to treat on the feet – you are, in effect, treating the lymphatic system while working the other parts of the body. In order to stimulate the thoracic duct, however, which runs in front of the spine in the area of the rib cage, it can be beneficial to work the reflex point for the corresponding part of the spine.

The body's lymphatic system and circulatory system (*see pp. 54-5*) are closely interconnected. The lymphatic system consists of a network of vessels of varying sizes distributed throughout the body. Its function is to trap any fluid that has escaped from the blood vessels and then return it to the body's blood supply. Once trapped, this fluid is known as lymph – a salty, straw-coloured substance like the liquid component of blood, but containing less protein. The system's other important function is to filter out bacteria and any other substances that could harm the body.

As has we have already seen when looking at the circulatory system, blood pressure forces oxygenated blood products through the very fine capillary walls to feed and nourish the cells of the surrounding tissue. Most of this liquid eventually find its way back into the capillaries; any that does not, however, is collected by the network of lymph vessels.

How the lymphatic system works

Think of the lymphatic system as a complicated network of waterways, streams, and tributaries. Instead of water, however, all of these channels carry lymph from many tiny vessels into a few larger channels. The largest of all of these is the thoracic duct, which runs up the length of the body just in front of the spine, or backbone. From the thoracic duct, lymph drains back into the blood supply near the left shoulder. The other major lymph vessel is known as the right lymphatic duct, which runs up through the right arm and shoulder. From this duct, lymph drains back into the bloodstream near the right shoulder.

Periodically, you may notice bumpy swellings in various parts of the body, most usually in the neck, armpits, and groin. These are inflamed lymph nodes that swell when the body's white blood cells congregate to fight and absorb harmful substances such as bacteria. Perhaps the best known of these lymph nodes are the tonsils.

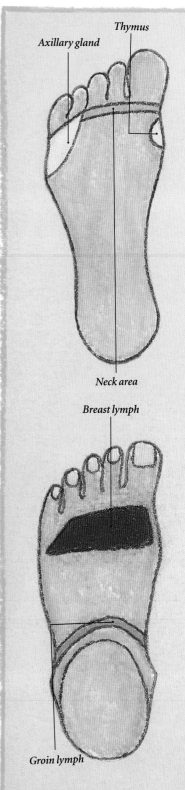

Axillary gland

Thymus

Neck area

Breast lymph

Groin lymph

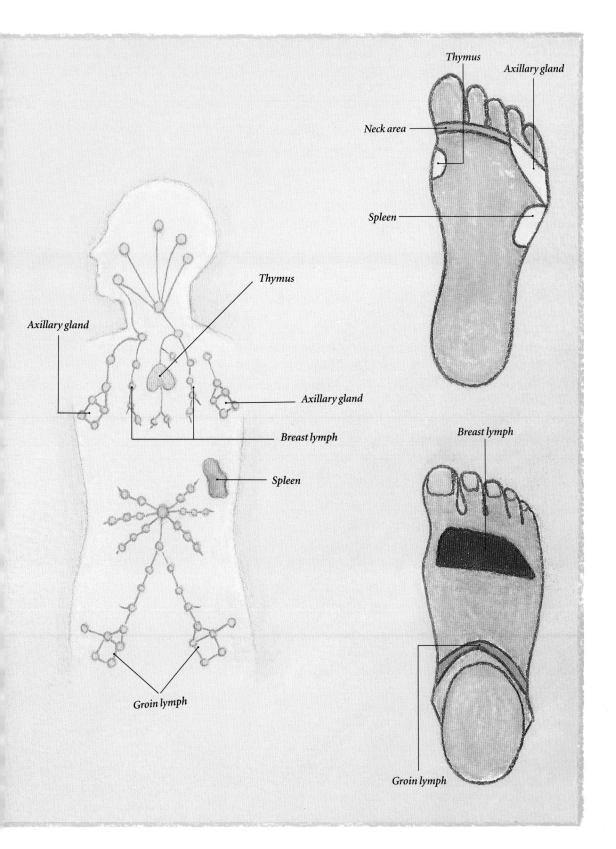

Thymus

Axillary gland

Neck area

Spleen

Thymus

Axillary gland

Axillary gland

Breast lymph

Spleen

Groin lymph

Breast lymph

Groin lymph

The Endocrine System

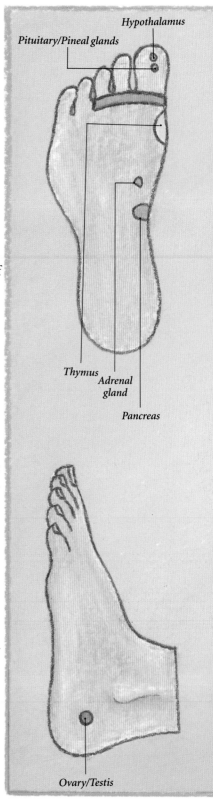

Hypothalamus

Pituitary/Pineal glands

Thymus
Adrenal gland

Pancreas

Ovary/Testis

Seeing that so many hormonal secretions have a direct or indirect effect in our mental and emotional wellbeing, the benefits of reflexology in treating the endocrine glands can potentially be extremely great. Reflexology seems to have the effect of regulating and balancing hormonal secretions – whether they are under- or overactive in their production – and, so, has had great success in treating both over- and underactive thyroid conditions, as well as depressive illnesses, and the all-too-common condition referred to as ME.

The endocrine glands are often referred to as ductless glands because their hormone secretions pass directly into the bloodstream. Each of these hormones is like a chemical messenger, manufactured by a particular gland with the specific purpose of influencing part of the body's activity, growth, or metabolism.

The glands making up the endocrine system are the pituitary gland, the thyroid gland, four parathyroids, two adrenal glands, the islets of Langerhans (found in the pancreas), the pineal gland (or body), the two ovaries in the female, and the two testes in the male (*see pp. 46-9*).

The pituitary gland and hypothalamus

The pituitary gland and the hypothalamus seem to act together as a single unit. The hypothalamus is not, in fact, classified as an endocrine gland, but as a part of the brain. It does, however, have a direct and controlling effect on the pituitary gland, which regulates the activity of most of the other endocrine glands in the body. This is why it is often referred to as the "master of the orchestra". The pituitary lies between the eyes and behind the nose, where it is protected by a strong arch of bone known as the *sella turcica*, or Turkish saddle.

The pineal gland

The pineal gland is a small reddish-brown body about ⅓in (1cm) long. It is located in the forebrain and is connected to the brain by a short stalk containing nerves, many of which terminate in the hypothalamus. The hormone secreted by the pineal gland is melatonin and there is now much evidence to suggest that the pineal gland has a direct influence on our moods and behaviour (*see p. 60*).

The thyroid gland

This gland, which also incorporates the parathyroids, is responsible for human growth and activity, metabolism, and the extraction of

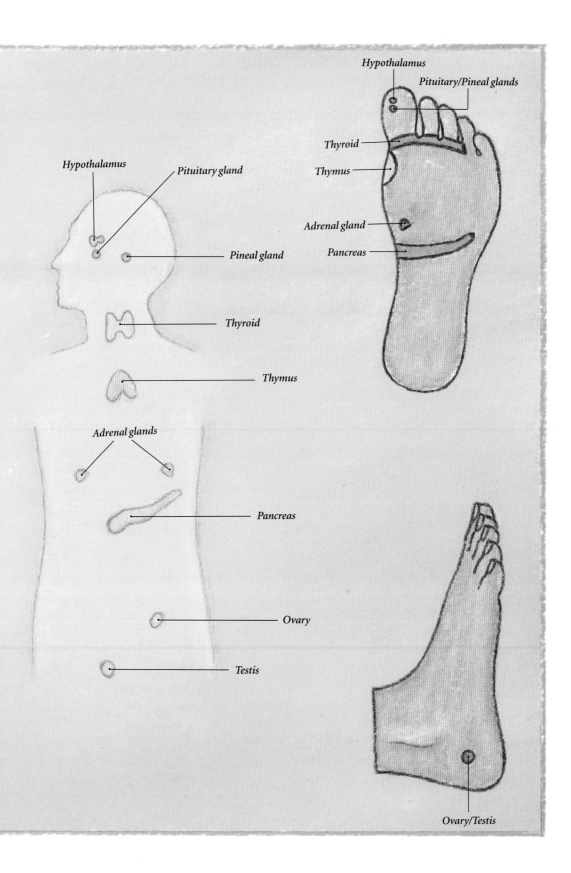

Hypothalamus

Pituitary gland

Pineal gland

Thyroid

Thymus

Adrenal glands

Pancreas

Ovary

Testis

Hypothalamus

Pituitary/Pineal glands

Thyroid

Thymus

Adrenal gland

Pancreas

Ovary/Testis

iodine from blood plasma. The thyroid has a great influence on our mental wellbeing. The thyroid gland also secretes the hormone thyroxine, a reduction of which can lead to severe neurotic tendencies in some people.

The islets of Langerhans
The cells making up the islets of Langerhans are found in irregularly distributed clusters throughout the pancreas. The hormonal secretions from these cell clusters pass directly into the veins of the pancreas and from there are distributed right around the body. A key function of the islets of Langerhans is the production of glucagon and of insulin, two hormones responsible for controlling the level of glucose in the bloodstream.

The pineal gland and behaviour
A recent study undertaken by a group of psychologists and psychiatrists has brought to light startling evidence of an apparent link between the pineal gland and the optic nerve.

The subjects of the study – Innuits living in the far north of Greenland – came to the attention of the researchers due to reported incidents of strange behavioural patterns among some individuals, including manic-depression, hysteria, and, in extreme cases, hysterical paralysis involving the loss of the use of one or more limbs. Since these behavioural problems occurred only during the winter, speculation arose that the long periods of semi-twilight and darkness that the north of Greenland is subjected to at that time of year might be responsible.

In order to test this speculation, a routine of ultraviolet ray treatment was administered to the area of the forehead corresponding to the position of the pineal gland of each test subject. After daily 20-minute sessions over a period of a month, about 90 per cent of those affected by behavioural problems reported complete recovery. It is now felt that ultraviolet light transmitted by the optic nerve had some sort of, as yet unexplained, corrective effect on the pineal gland and, hence, the rest of the brain.

Many people in less-extreme environments, where there is, nevertheless, a dramatic reduction in ultraviolet during winter, are familiar with the SAD (seasonal affective disorder) syndrome. Symptoms often include weight gain, mental and physical lethargy, and depression. It might be a reduction in sunlight that also accounts for the increase in admissions to psychiatric hospitals typical during the autumn and winter months. It is, therefore, not surprising to find great sensitivity in the big toe area of those suffering from depression, anxiety, and other stress-related conditions (*see pp. 14-17*).

Stress-related disorders

Stress and the endocrine system are closely associated. Therefore, the conditions that are going to be helped most by reflexology are tension- and stress-related disorders (*see pp. 14-17*). The reflex points that you need to work for the endocrine system are identical on both feet.

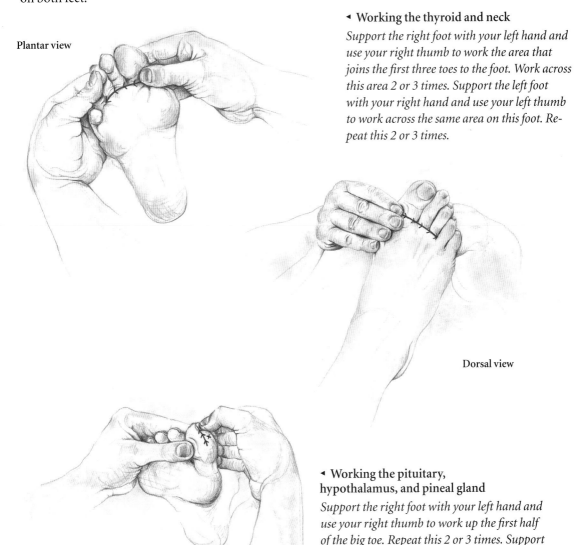

Plantar view

Dorsal view

◄ **Working the thyroid and neck**

Support the right foot with your left hand and use your right thumb to work the area that joins the first three toes to the foot. Work across this area 2 or 3 times. Support the left foot with your right hand and use your left thumb to work across the same area on this foot. Repeat this 2 or 3 times.

◄ **Working the pituitary, hypothalamus, and pineal gland**

Support the right foot with your left hand and use your right thumb to work up the first half of the big toe. Repeat this 2 or 3 times. Support the left foot with your right hand and use your left thumb to work up the first half of the big toe. Repeat this 2 or 3 times.

The Skeletal System

Back conditions are responsible for more working days lost than the common cold. All types of back pain, including sciatica, lumbago, disc lesions, and muscular spasms, should respond quickly to reflexology sessions, since this unique form of treatment relaxes the painful muscles and normalizes the functioning of the spine.

Basic construction

The human skeleton has three main functions: to provide support; to protect the internal organs; and, with the help of specialized groups of muscles, to provide the body with movement. The 206 bones that make up the skeleton can be divided into two broad groups. These are known as the axial and the appendicular groups. There is surprisingly little difference between a male and female skeleton except, as you would expect, that the bones of the male tend to be larger and heavier than those of the female. The axial skeleton is made up of the skull, spine, and rib cage, which gives the skeleton its basic framework on to which the appendicular limbs are joined via the pelvic and shoulder girdles. The pelvis is much heavier and stronger than the shoulder girdle. This is necessary because the pelvis has to support the full weight of the upper body.

The skeleton is built up of different types of bones: long bones, such as those from the hip to the knee and from the shoulder to the elbow; short bones, such as the fingers and toes; flat bones, represented by the cranium, scapula, and pelvic region; and irregularly shaped bones, such as the vertebrae found in the spine.

The vertebrae and ribs

The spinal column is similar in principle to a number of cotton reels threaded on to a length of rope. The spine is extremely flexible, being able to rotate, bend backward, forward, to the left, and to the right.

To achieve this degree of flexibility, the spine is a complicated construction made up of groups of vertebrae: 7 cervical vertebrae; 12 thoracic vertebrae; 5 lumbar vertebrae; 5 sacral vertebrae; and the 4 vertebrae that form the coccyx – a residual "tail".

The lumbar vertebrae are much denser and stronger than the thoracic vertebrae because of the extra weight the lumbar region has to bear – in fact, the whole weight of the upper body is supported from this region of the spine. The thoracic vertebrae are finer and have less density than the lumbar vertebrae, since they have less of a

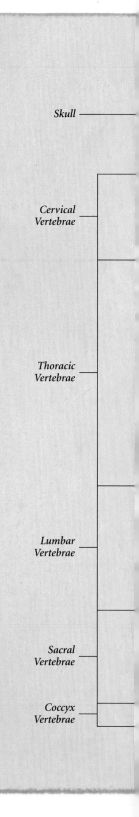

Skull

Cervical Vertebrae

Thoracic Vertebrae

Lumbar Vertebrae

Sacral Vertebrae

Coccyx Vertebrae

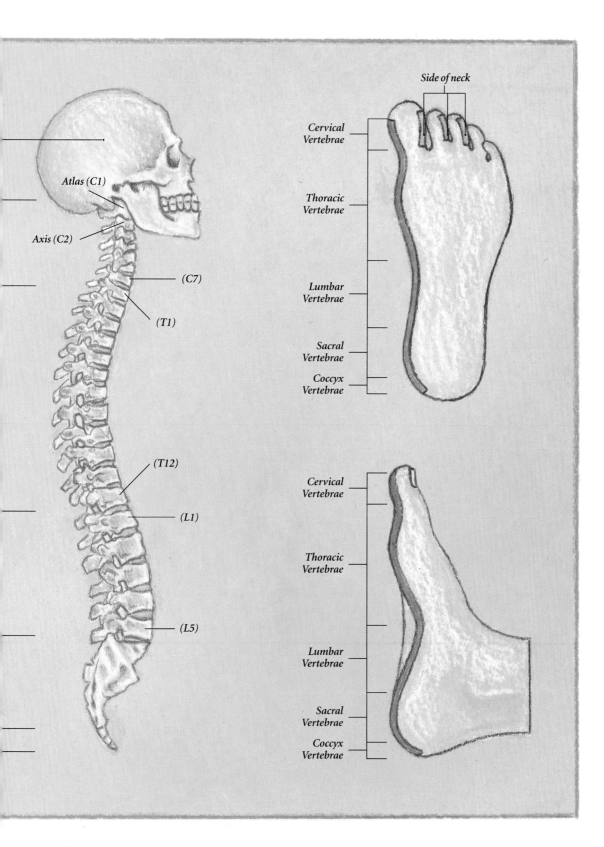

Atlas (C1)

Axis (C2)

(C7)

(T1)

(T12)

(L1)

(L5)

Side of neck

Cervical
Vertebrae

Thoracic
Vertebrae

Lumbar
Vertebrae

Sacral
Vertebrae

Coccyx
Vertebrae

Cervical
Vertebrae

Thoracic
Vertebrae

Lumbar
Vertebrae

Sacral
Vertebrae

Coccyx
Vertebrae

weight-bearing role to play and are mainly concerned with support-ing the structure of the rib cage. The cervical vertebrae are finer and lighter still, since they have to support only the weight of the skull. Two specialist vertebrae are found at the very top of the spine: the axis and atlas. The axis allows the head to rotate, while the atlas al-lows the head to nod up and down.

The thorax consists of 12 pairs of ribs that are connected to the thoracic vertebrae. The first 10 of these pairs are joined by cartilage to the sternum, which is a vertical bone in the centre of the chest, while the 2 lowest pairs are left unattached, or "floating".

The bones

All bones have a dense, outer layer and a spongy, inner centre. This type of arrangement makes them both strong and light. Bones also store calcium and phosphorus. The articulating surfaces of the bones are covered in cartilage to provide a smooth surface for the joints. Although bones have no nerve supplies, blood vessels enter them through the nutrient canal in order to feed and nourish the spongy central part.

Growth occurs in all of the bones but it is more obviously appar-ent in the long bones. All bones are formed from cartilage, which ossifies during the first few years of life. The only exceptions to this are the clavicle – the bones connecting the shoulder blades with the upper part of the breastbone – and parts of the skull.

The discs of the spine

The mobility of the vertebrae is due to the fact that the surface of each is covered with cartilage and the intervening space is filled with a thick disc of fibrous cartilage with a centre composed of soft, gelatinous tissue. These intervertebral discs act as shock absorbers for the spine. The movement between the individual vertebrae, with the exception of the axis and atlas, is only small, but the combined effect is considerable when taken overall.

Most of the skeleton's flexion and extension come from the cervical and lumbar regions of the spine; sideways bending is main-ly a function of the thoracic region; and twisting involves all of the vertebral column. The result of all these different types of movement is that the discs tend to wear out through the years, and they can become wafer thin.

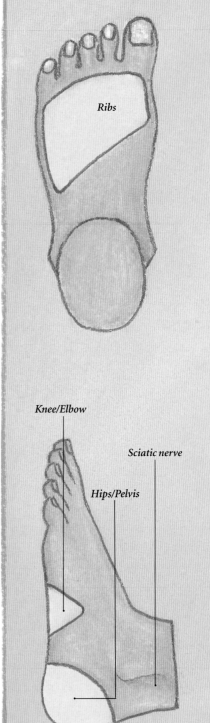

Ribs

Knee/Elbow

Sciatic nerve

Hips/Pelvis

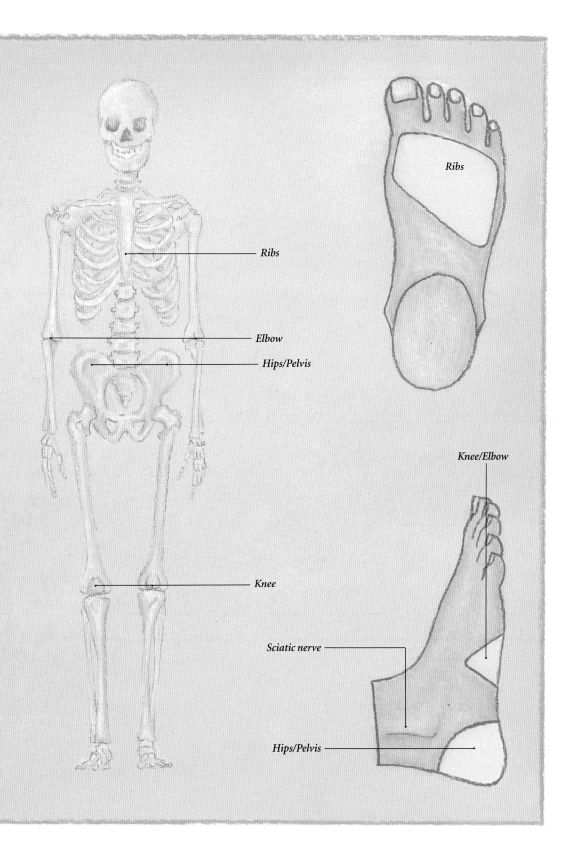

Ribs

Elbow

Hips/Pelvis

Knee

Ribs

Knee/Elbow

Sciatic nerve

Hips/Pelvis

The effects of wear on the skeleton

There are limitations in what reflexology can do to help with degenerative conditions of the spine, but generally it can at least offer some comfort by reducing pain and stiffness. Due to the constant movement of the joints, these areas are prone to many painful conditions. The reflex points for the skeleton are identical on both feet.

▾ **Working the coccyx**

Support the right foot with your right hand and apply pressure using the 4 fingers of your left hand. Repeat 2 or 3 times. Change your supporting hand for the left foot.

▾ **Working the hip/pelvis**

Support the right foot with your left hand and apply pressure using the 4 fingers of your right hand. Repeat 2 or 3 times. Change your supporting hand for the left foot and repeat the process.

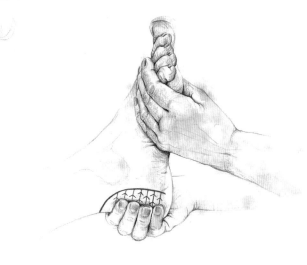

66

◂ **Working the spine**

Support the right foot with your left hand and use your right thumb to work the reflex points for the spine. Repeat 2 or 3 times. Repeat on the left foot, changing your supporting hand.

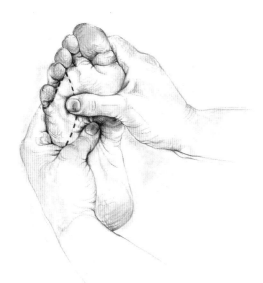

◄ Working the shoulder

Support the right foot with your left hand and work the shoulder area with your right thumb. Change your supporting hand and use your left thumb to work back across the area again. Support the left foot with your right hand and use your left thumb to work the shoulder area. Change your supporting hand and use your right thumb to work back over the area.

► Working the knee

Support the right foot with your right hand and use your left index finger to work the entire triangular-shaped area. Support the left foot with your left hand and use your right index finger to work the entire area.

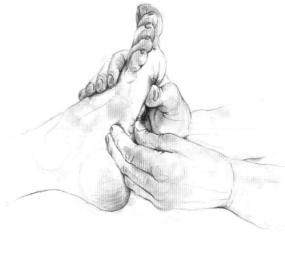

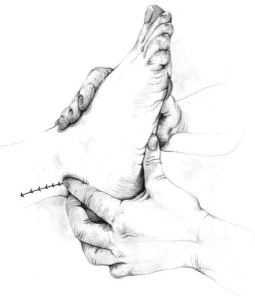

◄ Working the sciatic area

Support the right foot with your right hand and use the index and third fingers of your left hand to work up the area just behind the ankle for about 3in (7.5cm). Repeat 2 or 3 times. Change your supporting hand for the left foot and repeat this process with the index and third fingers of your right hand.

The Brain & Facial Areas

The brain together with the spinal cord comprise the body's central nervous system. The billions of nerve cells, called neurones, that make up the brain control consciousness, emotions, thought, movement, and a whole range of unconscious body functions.

Conditions that can affect the central nervous system range in severity from troublesome inflammations to life-threatening diseases. Reflexology can bring varying degrees of relief from such conditions as multiple sclerosis, Parkinson's disease, ear conditions, persistent ear, nose, and throat conditions in children, tired or strained eyes, and conjunctivitis. While it would not be possible to restore a multiple sclerosis sufferer who is wheelchair bound to an independently mobile state, good results have nevertheless been achieved in relieving the painful leg spasms associated with that condition. After treating upper-respiratory infections, it is quite common to hear people say that they spent the next day constantly blowing their noses, which can greatly benefit sinus conditions.

The structure of the brain

Stripped of its protective bony skull, the brain has the appearance of a very large, wrinkled walnut. In order to prevent the soft brain matter from being damaged by knocking against the inside of the skull, it is encased by two membranes, or meninges, filled with cerebrospinal fluid. The main parts of the brain are the cerebrum, the brain stem, and the cerebellum.

The cerebrum comprises about 70 per cent of the nervous system. It has a right cerebral hemisphere and a left cerebral hemisphere, which are connected by a mass of fibres. The cerebrum's wrinkled surface layer, or the cortex, contains the nerve cells that are commonly referred to as "grey matter", overlaying white matter made up of the nerve cell trunks. Different areas of the cerebrum deal with very specific functions: the motor cortex deals with voluntary movement; the sensory cortex with bodily sensations; the frontal lobe with personality; the occipital lobe with sight; and the middle of the brain is the hearing and speech centre.

The brain stem is a stalk of nerve fibres joining the spinal cord to the cerebellum and the cerebrum. Brain stem functions include the automatic and unconscious control of such activities as breathing and heart beat. The main functions of the cerebellum concern the coordination of muscles and the maintenance of bodily equilibrium.

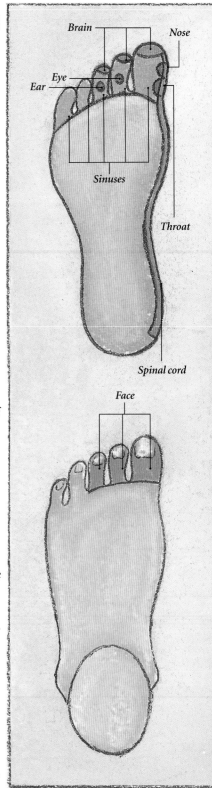

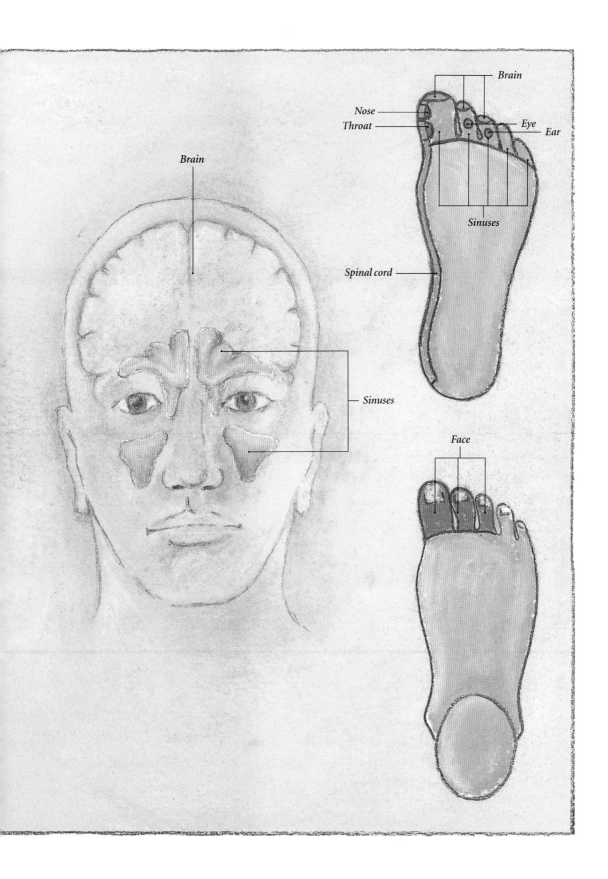

Brain

Nose

Throat

Brain

Eye

Ear

Sinuses

Spinal cord

Sinuses

Face

The ears

The internal structures of the ears enable us to hear and to maintain our balance. The human ear is able to distinguish sounds ranging in loudness between about 10 and 140 decibels. The distance between our ears helps the brain to locate the direction and source of sounds.

The ear has three distinct parts: the outer ear, the middle ear, and the inner ear. The outer ear consists of a flap of cartilage shaped to gather sound waves and direct them toward the meatus, or ear canal. The middle ear contains the ear drum and three small bones – the mallus (hammer), incus (anvil), and stapes (stirrup). The inner ear contains a fluid-filled coiled tube called the cochlea. This contains the nerve cells that connect with the auditory nerve that terminates in the brain. The organ of balance consists of three fluid-filled, U-shaped tubes set at right angles to each other. The tubes contain hairs that are sensitive to movement and special cells that are capable of sensing the positions of all parts of the body.

The eyes

Each eye looks looks like a ball of jelly about 1in (2.5cm) across. The sclera, or white, forms the outer layer of the eyeball, except for the transparent cornea at the front. Behind the cornea is the anterior chamber, containing a fluid called aqueous humour. This is separated from the posterior chamber by the lens. In front of the lens is a muscle, the iris. Light enters the eye through a central black hole, or pupil, and passes through the lens, which focuses an upside-down image on the special light- and colour-sensitive cells that form the retina. These cells stimulate the optic nerve at the back of each eye and messages are transmitted to the visual cortex of the brain. It is here that the overlapping fields of vision from both eyes are brought together to create our perception of a three-dimensional world.

The sinuses

Sinuses are air cavities in the bones of the face. As well as giving resonance to the voice, the sinuses act as filters for air breathed in through the nose, and their structure also helps to lighten the head and so reduce the weight loading on the spine. When infection of the sinuses occurs, facial pain is experienced and breathing through the nose can be extremely difficult or even impossible. Inflamed sinuses can also lead to a sensation of pain in the ears.

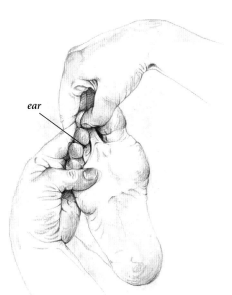

ear

◄ Working the eye and ear

Support the right foot with your left hand and use a gentle rotating movement of your right thumb on the second and third toes. Supporting the left foot with your right hand, use the same gentle, rotating movement of your left thumb on the second and third toes.

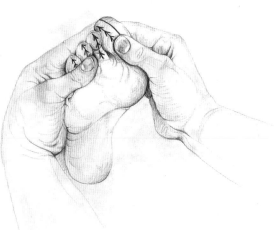

▶ Working the sinuses

Support the right foot in your left hand and use your right thumb to work the entire surface of the toe areas. Work from the medial to the lateral and, when you reach the little toe, change the supporting hand and use your left thumb to work from lateral to medial. Support the left foot in your right hand and use your left thumb to work the area of the toes. When you reach the little toe, change your supporting hand and use your right thumb to work back over the area.

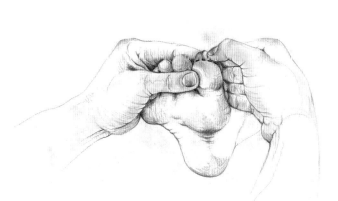

◄ Working the brain

Find the brain reflex points on the top of the first 3 toes. It is the same area on both feet. To work this area, apply a little pressure with your thumb on the top of the 3 toes on each foot. Use your right thumb on the right foot and your left thumb on the left foot.

The Muscular System

The body has three different types of muscle. The first is skeletal, or voluntary, muscle. This, together with the bones and tendons, is responsible for all types of conscious movement, as well as being involved in the automatic reactions known as reflexes. Voluntary muscles produce their effect by shortening in length, or contracting. Sudden, explosive contractions are necessary when you jump into the air, for example. These muscles make up about 25 per cent of your body weight.

The second type is known as smooth muscle, which is concerned with the involuntary movement of internal organs, such as the intestines and bladder. In smooth, or involuntary, muscle, each fibre is a long, spindly cell. This muscle is not under the conscious control of the brain but it is responsible for the types of muscular contractions required in such processes of digestion, where rhythmic squeezing of the intestines moves food through the system.

The third type of muscle is cardiac muscle, which makes up the majority of the heart. Cardiac muscle has a structure similar to that of voluntary muscle, but its fibres are short and thick and form a dense mesh.

Since muscles are distributed throughout the entire body, there are no special reflexology procedures to adopt in helping muscular aches and pains. You are, in fact, working the muscular system of the body as you work through a treatment session.

How muscles work

Skeletal muscle fibres are activated by motor nerves in the spinal cord. These nerves branch as they enter a skeletal muscle, so that each branch makes contact with a different muscle fibre. Individual muscles can act only to shorten, not lengthen, the distance between two attachment points – they can pull but not push. For movement in the opposite direction, another muscle must be used. For example, the biceps on top of the upper arm can flex the elbow, but the triceps under the upper arm are responsible for extending the limb.

Smooth muscle is also supplied with motor nerves. However, instead of one motor nerve making contact with an individual muscle fibre, stimulation spreads in a wave over several muscle fibres. This wave-like action helps in moving food through the intestines, for example.

Cardiac muscle contracts when pulses under the control of the autonomic nervous system emanate from special pacemaker tissue in the heart. These pulses pass through the heart about 70 times every minute, causing the heart to beat in a regular way.

The Solar Plexus

Just behind the stomach wall lies the network of nerves known as the solar plexus. Reflexology treatment of the solar plexus region occurs automatically every time you treat the digestive system on the left-hand side of the body (*see pp. 42-5*), so you will be making contact with this area reasonably frequently. This is all to the good, since it does create a general feeling of wellbeing and relaxation in the person being treated.

It is usual to pick up a lot sensitivity in the reflex points corresponding to the solar plexus when you are treating somebody who is under emotional stress and strain. The feelings of nervousness and anxiety we are all familiar with also come from this area as signals in the form of "butterflies in the stomach".

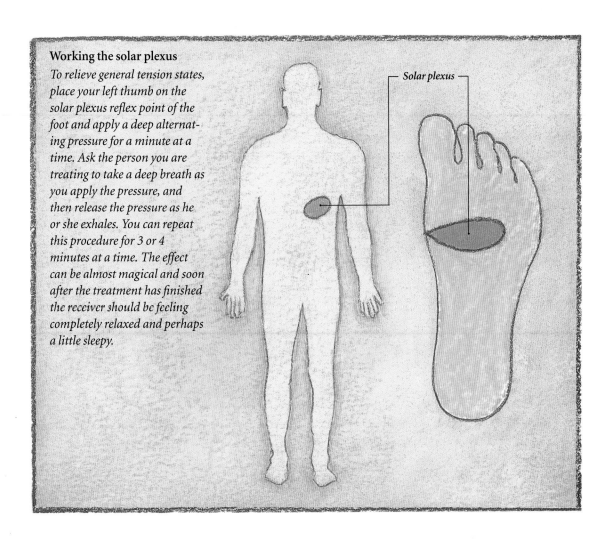

Working the solar plexus

To relieve general tension states, place your left thumb on the solar plexus reflex point of the foot and apply a deep alternating pressure for a minute at a time. Ask the person you are treating to take a deep breath as you apply the pressure, and then release the pressure as he or she exhales. You can repeat this procedure for 3 or 4 minutes at a time. The effect can be almost magical and soon after the treatment has finished the receiver should be feeling completely relaxed and perhaps a little sleepy.

Solar plexus

The Urinary System

The types of problem related to the urinary system that can be helped by reflexology include stress incontinence, cystitis, which mainly affects women, and pain from renal colic. High blood pressure is firmly linked to renal function, and a lowering of blood pressure can also be brought about by reflexology.

The body's urinary system is made up of two kidneys, two ureter tubes, and a bladder, which is controlled by a sphincter muscle.

The kidneys

The kidneys are important organs designed to filter out impurities from the bloodstream and so prevent poisons building up to dangerous levels. These bean-shaped organs are located behind the stomach, one each side of the spine. A single kidney contains more than a million nephrons, which are tiny blood filtration units.

Urine, the waste product of filtration, collects in the kidney's pelvis. Blood for processing enters the kidney through the medulla – the innermost part of the organ – from the renal artery. Once filtered, the liquid continues through a small tube, or tubule, surrounded by capillaries. These tiny capillaries reabsorb most of the water and useful chemicals and the treated blood leaves the kidney via the renal vein. Meanwhile, urine – the waste products left behind in the kidneys – leaves through its respective ureter tube and collects in the urinary bladder. One pair of kidneys can process up to 42 gallons (190 litres) of blood in a single day. Urine output drops off while you sleep or when you are perspiring heavily and rises when you drink more liquid than usual. Together, the kidneys are about the same size as the heart.

The bladder

The bladder is a hollow, muscular bag found just behind the hip bone, or pubis. A broad tube, called the urethra, opens from the bottom of the bladder. A ring of muscle, the urethral sphincter, normally keeps this outlet firmly closed.

An empty bladder lies flat inside the body, while a fully inflated one can hold approximately a pint of urine. As urine drips from the two ureter tubes, the walls of the bladder relax in order to accommodate the liquid. Once about a cupful of urine has collected, nerves signal the brain and urge urination. As the urethral sphincter muscles relax and the walls of the bladder contract, urine is forced out of the urethra.

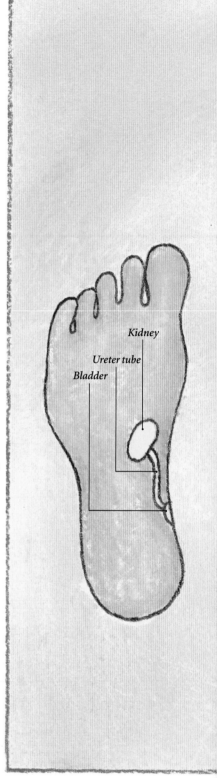

Kidney

Ureter tube
Bladder

Treating the urinary system

The reflex points for the urinary system are identical on both feet, with half the bladder reflex points being found on the medial side of the right foot and the other half on the medial side of the left foot.

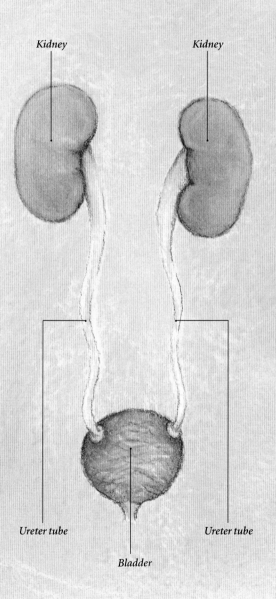

Kidney   *Kidney*

Ureter tube   *Ureter tube*

Bladder

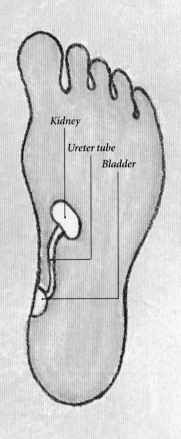

Kidney

Ureter tube

Bladder

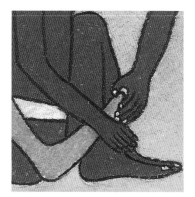

Chapter Five

Treating the Feet

Before starting a reflexology foot session (*see pp. 80-7*), it is important to make sure that the receiver is relaxed. The feet relaxation exercises opposite, and continuing on pages 78-9, are designed to help the receiver gain maximum benefit from any reflexology treatment. The first step, however, is to settle the receiver comfortably, either in a reclining-type chair or stretched out on a sun lounger (*see p. 38*). If the receiver is in any way uncomfortable, tension will soon start to build up. This will be transmitted through to the feet, making them harder to work on and the treatment generally less beneficial.

A reflexology session should take about 50 minutes the first time, but as you become more experienced you should be able to trim 5 to 10 minutes off this total. If any of the reflex points are very sensitive, work over them again (*see also pp. 98-135 for specific complaints*).

Relaxation techniques for the feet
The following relaxation exercises are designed to make the feet supple and flexible. They may also prove important if a specific system (*see pp. 42-75*) is causing particular sensitivity in the feet, thus making them difficult to treat. Those new to reflexology may also find these exercises valuable as a training routine, since they quickly get you accustomed to handling the feet properly and to maintaining constant contact with the feet throughout a session.

For each exercise, start on the right foot and then repeat the same routine on the left. You need spend only about 10 to 15 seconds on each exercise per foot.

Important
You may be tempted to apply oil or creams to the receiver's feet before starting a session. This, however, makes good contact with the foot extremely difficult. If necessary, lightly dust the feet with talcum powder in order to give yourself a good, dry surface on which to work.

Feet Relaxation Exercises

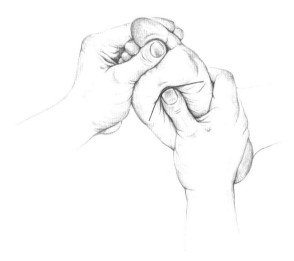

Starting with the right foot, place your right thumb on the beginning of the diaphragm line. Move your thumb outward, toward the lateral side of the foot. At the same time, bend the toes downward on to your left thumb. Repeat this exercise for the left foot.

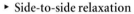

▸ **Side-to-side relaxation**
While supporting the foot at the top, use a side-to-side rocking movement with both hands to relax the foot. Begin with the right foot and repeat the exercise for the left foot.

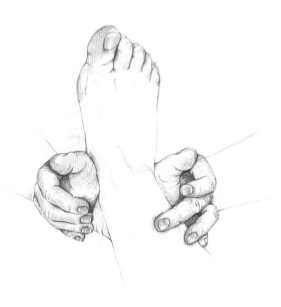

◂ **Ankle freeing**
This exercise is extremely effective for those with stiff ankles. Start with the right foot and, using both hands, gently rock the foot from side to side. Repeat this exercise for the left foot.

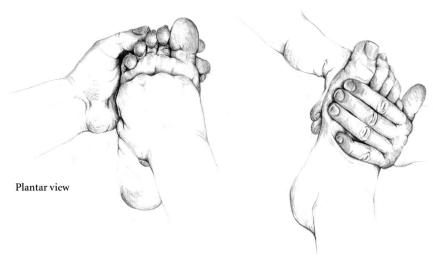

Dorsal view

Plantar view

▲ Metatarsal kneading

Begin on the right foot and place your right fist on the sole of the right foot. Place your left hand over the front of the foot. Then, use a pushing movement from the plantar side combined with a squeezing movement from the dorsal side. Both movements must be in harmony with each other. Repeat this exercise for the left foot.

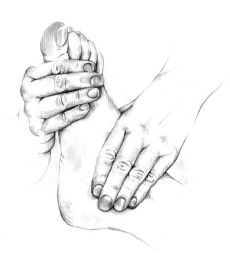

◄ Overgrip

Place your left hand over the top of the right ankle, making sure that the thumb of your left hand is on the outside edge of the foot. Turn the foot in an inward direction, using a light circling movement. Repeat this exercise for the left foot. This exercise is very effective for any swelling of the ankles.

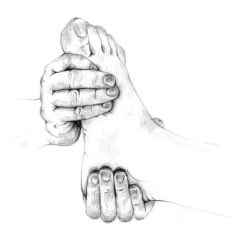

◂ Undergrip

Start with the right foot and place your left hand under the ankle as a support. Your thumb must be on the lateral side of the foot. Turn the foot in an inward direction, using a light circling movement. Repeat this exercise for the left foot.

▸ Foot moulding

Sandwich the right foot between your two hands, supporting it from the lateral edge. Gently rotate both hands, making a movement like that of the wheels of a train. Repeat this exercise for the left foot.

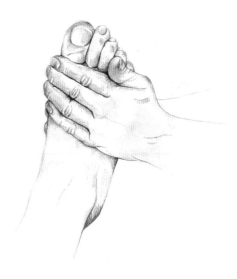

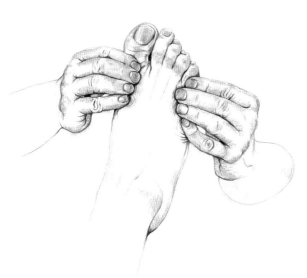

◂ Relaxing the rib cage

Starting on the right foot, press in with both of your thumbs and use all the fingers of both of your hands to creep around to the dorsal side of the foot. Repeat this exercise for the left foot.

The Basic Foot Session

▶ **Working the lung/breast**

Plantar view: Supporting the right foot with your left hand, work up the area from the very base of the diaphragm line to where the toes join the foot. Dorsal view: Make a fist with your left hand and press it into the plantar side side of the right foot, and use your right index finger to work down the grooves in the foots. Repeat these steps on the left foot.

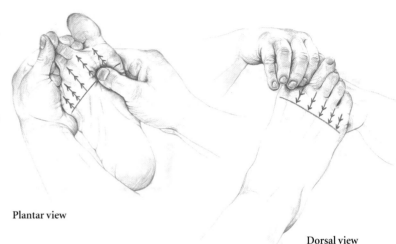

Plantar view

Dorsal view

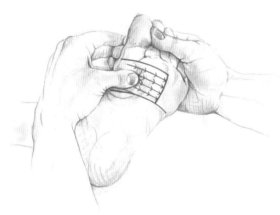

◀ **Working the heart**

The reflex points for the heart are found only on the left foot. Supporting the top of the left foot with your right hand and use your left thumb to work over the area from the medial edge of the foot. After working the area, use the diaphragm-relaxation exercise (see p. 77).

▶ **Working the sinuses**

Supporting the right foot with your left hand, use your right thumb to work up all 5 toes. Start at the very base of each and use a small, creeping movement to contact the entire surface of each toe. Repeat this for the left foot, using your right hand for support and left thumb to work the toes.

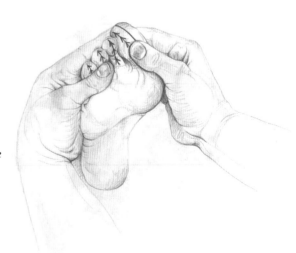

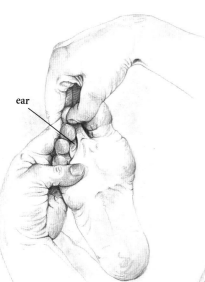

ear

◄ Working the eye and ear

To treat the eye, support the right foot with your left hand and place your right thumb directly under the first bend of the joint of the second toe. Use a small rotating movement in a clockwise direction. Use the same support and rotate technique on the third toe to treat the ear. Change your supporting hand and thumb to treat the left foot.

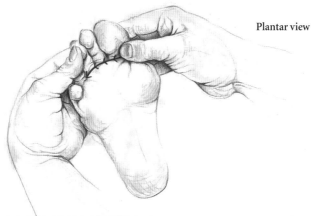

Plantar view

► Working the neck and thyroid

Plantar view: Support the right foot with your left hand and use your right thumb to work across the bases of the first 3 toes. Dorsal view: Use your right index finger to work across the bases of the first 3 toes. For the left foot, use your right hand for support, your left thumb for the plantar, and your left index finger for the dorsal.

Dorsal view

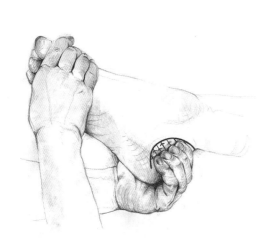

◄ Working the coccyx

Holding the right foot in an outward direction (away from the body) with your right hand, use the 4 fingers of your left hand to creep around the medial edge of the foot. To treat the left foot, use your right hand for support and the fingers of your left hand to creep around the medial edge.

▶ Working the hip and pelvis

Holding the right foot in an outward direction (away from the body) with your left hand, use all 4 fingers of your right hand to creep around the lateral edge of the foot. To treat the left foot, use your right hand for support and the fingers of your left hand to creep around the lateral edge.

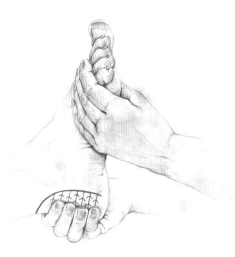

◀ Working the spine

Holding the right foot in an outward direction (away from the body) with your left hand, use your right thumb to work up the medial edge of the foot. To work the left foot, use your right hand for support and your left thumb to work up the medial edge. After working the spine, use the ankle-freeing exercise (see p. 77).

▶ Working the brain

Supporting the right foot with your left hand, work over the top of the big toe with your right thumb. To work the left foot, use your right hand to support the foot and your left thumb to work the big toe.

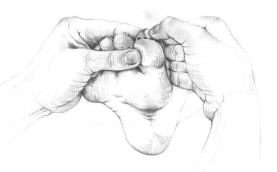

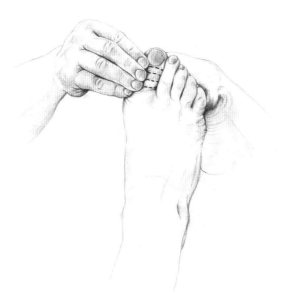

◄ **Working the face**
*Make a fist with your left hand and push it
into the plantar side of the right foot. Then
use your right index finger to work the
area on the dorsal side of the big toe. To
treat the left foot, make a fist with your
right hand and use your left index finger
to work the area on the dorsal side of the
big toe.*

▶ **Working the shoulder**
*Support the right foot with your left hand
and work the area just under the fifth toe
with your right thumb. For the left foot,
use your right hand for support and your
left thumb to work the reflex point.*

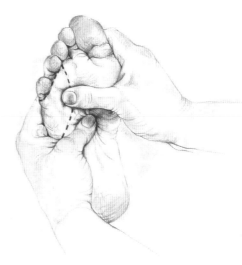

◄ **Working the knee and elbow**
*Support the right foot with your right hand
and use your left index finger to work the triangular area on the lateral side of the foot.
To treat the left foot, use your left hand for support and your right index finger to work the
same area on the lateral side of the foot.*

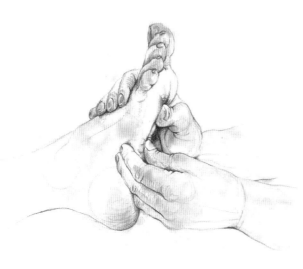

▶ **Working the sciatic nerve**

Supporting the right foot with your right hand, use your left index finger to work the area directly behind the ankle bone. Proceed up the leg for about 3in (7.5cm). To treat the left foot, use your left hand for support and your right index finger to work the area behind the ankle bone and leg.

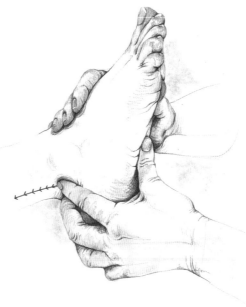

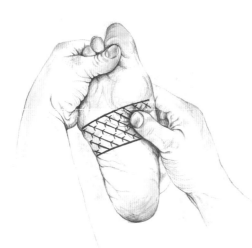

◀ **Working the liver**

The reflex points for the liver are found only on the right foot. Support the right foot with your left hand and use your right thumb to work the area indicated.

▶ **Working the stomach and pancreas**

The reflex points for these areas are found only on the left foot. Support the left foot with your right hand and use your left thumb to work the areas indicated.

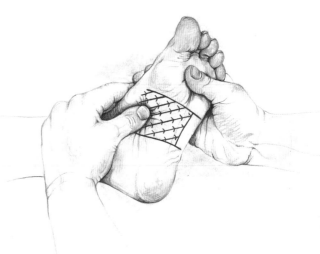

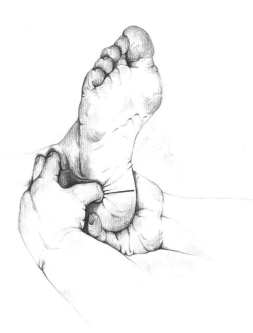

◄ **Working the ileocecal valve**

The reflex point for the ileocecal valve is found only on the right foot. Support the heel of the right foot with your right hand and use the hooking-out technique (see p. 39) with your left thumb.

(see p. 39)

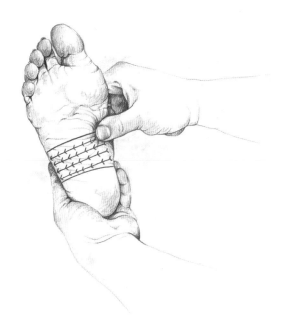

► **Working the intestines (ascending and transverse colons and small intestines)**

The reflex points for these areas are found only on the right foot. Support the right foot with your left hand and use your right thumb to work the area to the base of the heel.

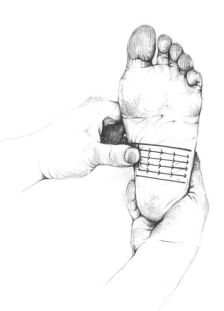
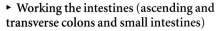

◄ **Working the intestines (transverse and descending colon)**

The reflex points for these area are found on the left foot. Support the left foot with your right hand and work across the foot to the base of the heel with your left thumb.

▶ Working the bladder

Supporting the right right foot with your left hand, use your right thumb to work on the soft, rather puffy area on the medial edge of the foot. To work on the left foot, change your supporting hand and use your left thumb to work on the same area.

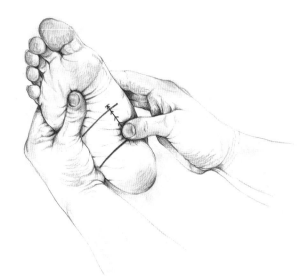

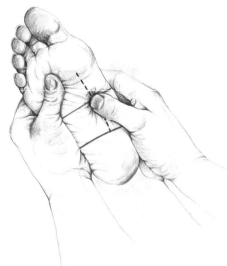

◀ Working the ureter

Supporting the right foot with your left hand, use your right thumb to work the area. When working on the left foot, use the same technique, but change your supporting hand and use your left thumb to work the area.

Note: Take care not to work directly on the ligament line. Always apply pressure on the medial side of this line, otherwise you will cause a lot of discomfort for the receiver.

▶ Working the kidneys

Supporting the right foot with your left hand, rotate the foot around your right thumb. For the left foot, change your supporting hand and rotate the foot around your left thumb. In most people, the kidney reflex point tends to be more sensitive than most, and so this technique causes least discomfort.

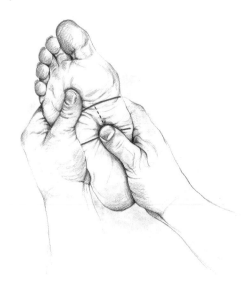

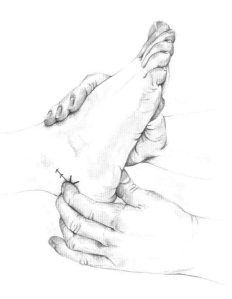

◄ **Working the ovaries/testes**

Supporting the right foot with your right hand, tilt the foot in an outward direction and use your left index finger to work the area indicated. For the left foot, change supporting hand and use your right index finger to work the area.

▶ **Working the uterus/prostate**

Support the right foot with your left hand and use your right index finger to work from the tip of the heel to the ankle bone. For the left foot, change your supporting hand and use your left index finger to work the same area.

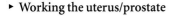

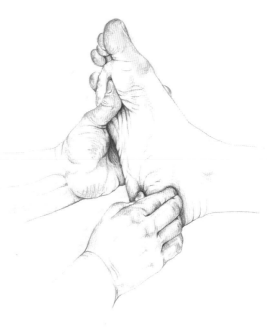

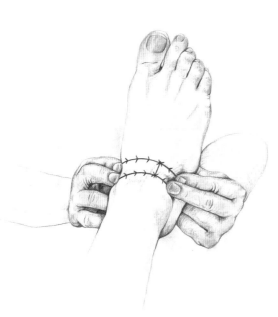

◄ **Working the fallopian tubes/vas deferens**

Using both thumbs, press into the sole of the foot while working over the top of the foot with the index fingers of both hands. Repeat this same technique for the left foot.

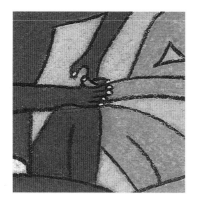

Chapter Six

Treating the Hands

The most direct and powerful benefits of reflexology come from applying pressure to the reflex points found on and around the feet (*see pp. 76-87*). However, since two people are required – the giver and the receiver – foot reflexology is not practicable as a self-help therapy. Looking back at the maps of the hands (*see pp. 32-5*), you can see that all the reflex points corresponding to the body's systems are also present on the hands and wrists. Thus, hand reflexology can be used at any time – at your place of work or at home – to help relieve tension or stress or to treat a specific ailment (*see pp. 98-135*) between foot reflexology sessions.

The relaxation exercises and hand session
Although hand reflexology is recommended primarily as a self-help technique, there may be instances when it is used instead of working on the feet. For people who have had their feet amputated or severely damaged in some way, for example, hand reflexology can be given by another person. In these circumstances, the hand relaxation exercises opposite and continuing on pages 90-1 will be of benefit in relaxing the hands before undertaking a full hand session (*see pp. 92-7*). For each exercise, start on the right hand and then repeat the same routine on the left. About 10 to 15 seconds on each exercise per hand is sufficient.

Important
Do not apply any oil or cream to the hands as a prelude to the relaxation exercises or session. This will make good contact with the skin impossible. If necessary, lightly dust the hands with talcum powder before starting.

Hand Relaxation Exercises

These relaxation exercises are possible only if you have a helper, since two free hands are required. They are, however, by no means central to a successful hand reflexology session so you should not worry if they are omitted. If you do have a helper, the exercises can be carried out in any order.

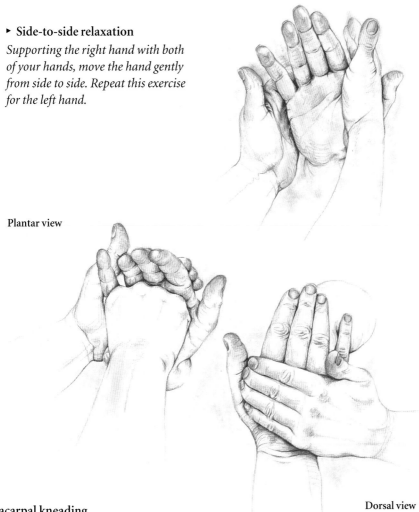

▶ **Side-to-side relaxation**
Supporting the right hand with both of your hands, move the hand gently from side to side. Repeat this exercise for the left hand.

Plantar view

Dorsal view

▶ **Metacarpal kneading**
Supporting the right hand with your left hand, make a fist with your right hand and use it to knead the receiver's palm. Repeat this exercise for the left hand, using your right hand as a support and making a fist with your left hand.

▸ Diaphragm relaxation

This exercise is excellent for relaxing the respiratory system. Working on the right hand, place your left thumb on the diaphragm line and gently bend the fingers over on to your thumb. Move your left thumb along this line from the medial to the lateral edge. Repeat this exercise for the left hand.

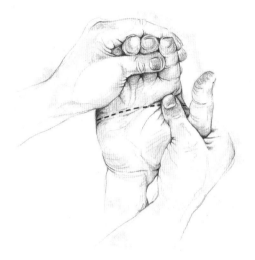

◂ Wrist freeing

Support the right hand just in front of the wrist with the heels of both your hands and rock the hand from side to side. Repeat this exercise for the left hand.

▸ Undergrip

Support the right hand by placing your left hand under the wrist, and use your right hand to turn the hand inward. Repeat this exercise for the left hand.

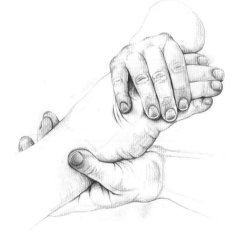

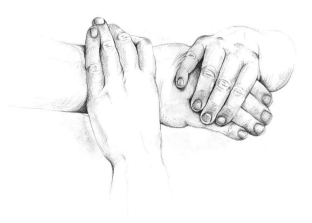

◄ Overgrip

Support the right hand by placing your left hand over the top of the wrist, and use your right hand to turn the hand inward. Repeat this exercise for the left hand.

◄▼ Hand moulding

Cradle the right hand between both of your hands, and then gently rotate your hands making a movement like that of the wheels of a train. Repeat this exercise for the left hand.

Dorsal view

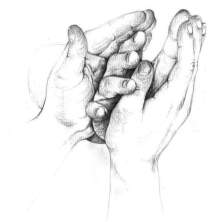

Plantar view

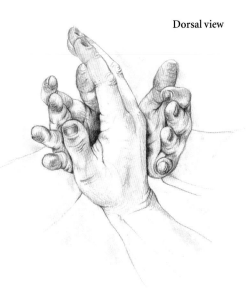

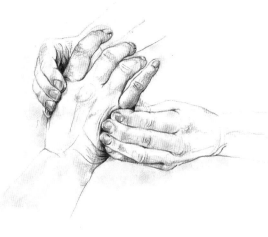

◄ Relaxing the rib cage

Working on the right hand, press in with the thumbs of both of your hands and creep around the dorsal side of the hand with the 4 free fingers of each hand. Repeat this exercise for the left hand.

The Basic Hand Session

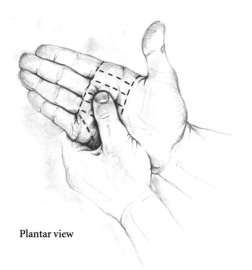

Plantar view

◄ ▼ Working the lung

Place your left thumb on the diaphragm line of your right hand. Work up in straight lines to where the fingers join the hand. On the dorsal side, place your left index finger on the join of the fingers to the hand and work down for about an 1in (2.5cm). Repeat this procedure for your left hand.

Dorsal view

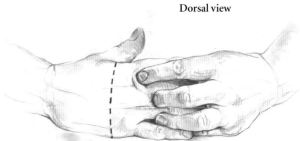

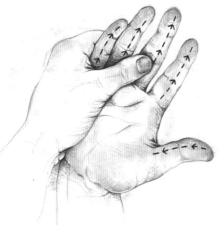

◄ Working the sinuses

Starting on your right hand, use the thumb of your left hand to work the reflex points in the directions of the arrows shown. Repeat this procedure for your left hand.

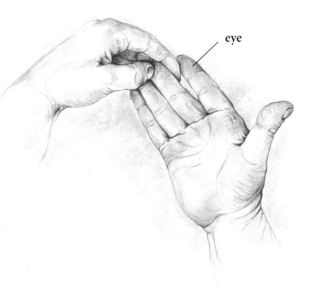

eye

► Working the eye and ear

Using your left thumb, apply pressure to the first bend of the index finger of your right hand, using a rotating movement (see p. 39). Use the same technique for the eye reflex point on the bend of the first joint of your third finger. Repeat this procedure for your left hand.

▼ ▶ Working the neck and thyroid gland

Using the thumb of your left hand, work the reflex points found at the base of the thumb and first 2 fingers of your right hand. The thyroid gland reflex point is at the base of the thumb, but by working on the bases of the next 2 fingers as well, you will be able to relieve neck tension. Repeat this procedure for your left hand.

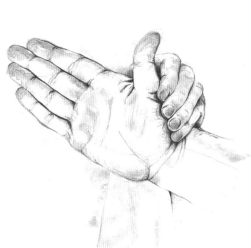

Plantar view

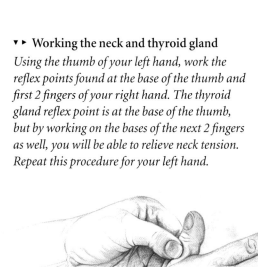

Dorsal view

▶ Working the coccyx

To work this reflex point, apply pressure from the 4 fingers of your left hand to the area just in front of the thumb on the medial side of your right hand. Repeat this procedure for your left hand.

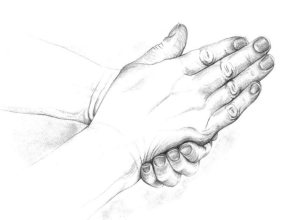

◄ Working the hip and pelvis

Apply pressure from the 4 fingers of your left hand around the lateral side of your right hand. Repeat this procedure for your left hand.

▶ **Working the spine**

To contact the reflex points for the spine on your right hand, work along the line indicated with your left thumb. For your left hand, use your right thumb to work over the corresponding area on that hand.

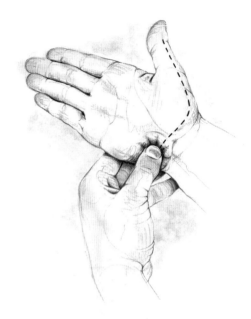

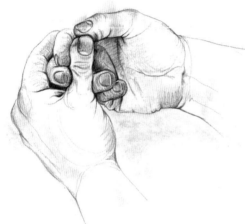

◀ **Working the brain**

To work the right side of the brain, apply pressure with left thumb directly to the top of your right thumb. Repeat this procedure for your left hand.

▶ **Working the shoulder**

To work the right shoulder, apply pressure to the area indicated on your right hand using your left thumb. Repeat this procedure on your left hand to contact the reflex points for your left shoulder.

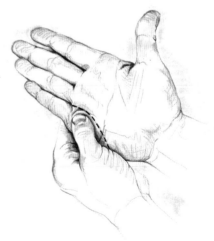

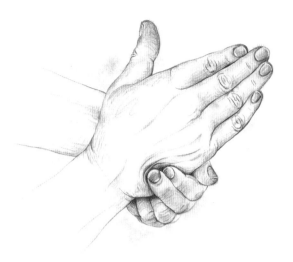

◄ **Working the knee and elbow**
On he right hand, work out the small triangular area using the fingers of your left hand. Repeat this procedure for the left hand.

► **Working the stomach, pancreas, and spleen**
The reflex points for these parts of the body are found only on the left hand. Use your right thumb to work over the areas indicated on your left palm. In the same area of the right hand you will contact the reflex point for the liver.

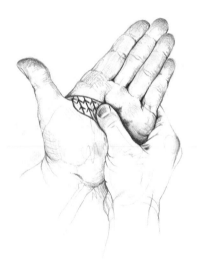

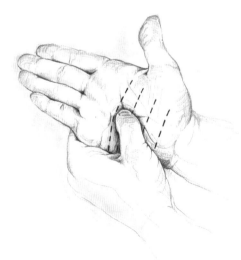

◄ **Working the ascending transverse and descending colon**
Using your left thumb, work across the palm of your right hand in the areas indicated. Repeat this procedure for your left hand.

▶ Working the bladder

Using your left thumb, apply pressure to the fleshy pad just below the thumb of your right hand. Repeat this procedure for your left hand.

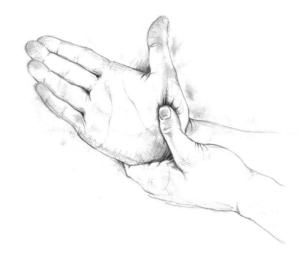

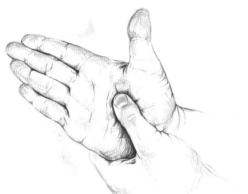

◀ Working the ureter

Working on the right hand with your left thumb, continue from the bladder section toward the base of your index finger. Repeat this procedure for your left hand.

▶ Working the kidney

Continuing upward from the line referred to above in working the ureter, you will find the reflex point for your kidney where your thumb joins the hand. Work the point with the thumb of your left hand, and repeat this procedure for your left hand.

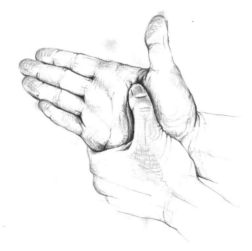

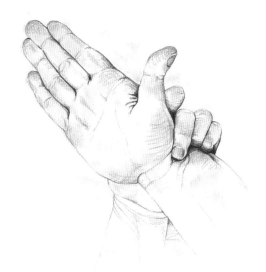

◄ Working the uterus/prostate

Use the third finger of your left hand to contact and work the reflex points on the area of your right wrist below the thumb. Repeat this procedure for your left hand.

► Working the ovaries/testes

Use the third finger of your left hand to contact and work the reflex point just in front of your right wrist bone. Repeat this procedure for your left hand.

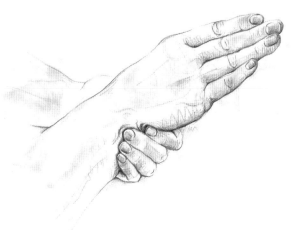

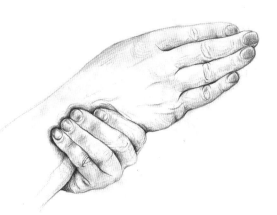

◄ Working the fallopian tubes/vas deferens

Using pressure from all 4 fingers of your left hand, work over the area on the lateral side of your right hand. Repeat this procedure for your left hand.

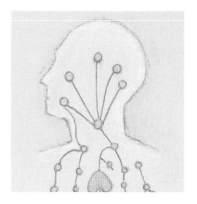

Chapter Seven
Treating Specific Ailments

When you become involved in any field of complementary medicine, such as reflexology, you will inevitably be more successful in your endeavours if you gain some understanding of how the body works, how the individual parts interact, one with another, to make up the whole being (*see pp. 40-75*).

Although the aim of reflexology is to balance and harmonize the way the body works, don't fall into the way of thinking that disease can somehow be eradicated. Disease is an integral part of living and has been with us from the very earliest of times. In our relatively recent, recorded history, we know of the Black Death, the bubonic plague that swept through Europe during the 14th century. It is estimated that up to 50 per cent of the population of England died of the plague during an 11-year period. Other killers of the past include diphtheria, tuberculosis, and polio, while today we are more likely to succumb to the modern killers – heart disease or cancer.

Unfortunately, we all inherit weaknesses or predispositions to certain diseases in our genetic coding. For example, you may have a tendency to arthritis, allergies, or migraine – even frequent back problems are more common in some families than in others. It is not possible to change our genetic structure, but we can change the way we treat and respect our bodies.

Targeting problem areas
The aim of reflexology is to improve and strengthen the weak areas of the body that are causing the condition or symptoms. This is

achieved by targeting the problem areas through the reflex points found on or around the feet or hands. These reflex points correspond to every part or system in the body (*see pp. 40-75*).

Looking beneath the surface

Sometimes, however, it is not enough to work just on the reflex point for, say, the head if you have a headache or migraine. The pain you are experiencing may merely be the manifestation of an underlying condition. In this example, the root cause of the headache could be a build-up of tension in the region of the neck or even an allergic reaction to certain types of food. If you suspect this to be the case, then the reflexology treatment will be more beneficial if it is concentrated on the reflex points corresponding to the neck or the digestive system. Certainly you should not ignore the painful area itself, and so some work on the head reflex point would probably help to ease the immediate discomfort you are experiencing.

How many times have you come home tired from work and said to your partner that some person or other has been a real pain in the neck during the day, and later that evening you have developed a splitting headache? There is often more than a grain of truth in these expressions we use and, if you are alert, you will start to develop an insight into the cause-and-effect element of many of the common ailments that afflict us from time to time. If, though, you have any symptoms that worry you or that persist, you should not hesitate in consulting your family doctor. Reflexology is intended to complement orthodox medical care, not supplant it in any way.

Body maintenance

It would be ideal if we all gave our bodies the same level of regular and routine preventive care and service that we do to our cars, for example, but few of us ever do. Typically, we ignore the early warning signs that all is not well, such as aches and pains or just feeling below par and "under the weather", and wait until we fall prey to some unpleasant condition that may require weeks or even months of reflexology treatment to put right again. Remember that it only takes a small stone to trigger a landslide.

It is not unusual to find that after a reflexology treatment session your condition seems a little worse than before you started. This reaction should not persist for more than a day and it is very rare for it to continue beyond 24 hours. The reasons for this type of reaction, particularly when treating problems such as migraine, asthma, bowel complaints, and other organic conditions, is that reflexology stimulates the organs of elimination – the liver, lungs, kidneys, lymphatic system, and the bowel. This stimulation causes toxins to be released into the bloodstream as a prelude to their removal from the body. The result is that short-term symptoms of headaches, increased urination and bowel movements, or sometimes a rash are not uncommon and should not be the cause of alarm, unless they persist.

Although it sounds contradictory, these are in fact healing signs and indicate that the body is eliminating waste products and toxins before starting to repair itself. Nature requires a clean slate on which to start the process of rebuilding, and reflexology can be an instrumental part of that process.

It is a good idea to drink plenty of bottled mineral water following a reflexology treatment session. The water assists in flushing out your system and may help to limit the type of reaction you could experience. Just bear in mind that these reactions are a positive sign and that they are nothing to be bothered about. They are a tangible indication that the reflexology treatment is working and stimulating the different systems in your body, and that your body is responding as it should.

Adopting the right approach

The most noticeable reactions of the type described above are likely to occur after your initial reflexology treatment; subsequent sessions are unlikely to give rise to any troublesome symptoms. But don't expect reflexology to bring about an instantaneous release from whatever complaint prompted you to seek help in the first place. Your expectations need to be realistic, so bear in mind that progress will, in most cases, be gradual. Week by week you will start to feel progressively better until, by about the sixth or seventh weekly session, you should experience a very definite improvement in your general health condition.

Although this chapter of the book concentrates on treating specific ailments, good reflexology practice dictates that each treatment session should start with a series of relaxation exercises for the feet or, if the feet cannot be used for some reason, the hands. You will find these at the beginning of the relevant treatment chapters (*see pp. 76-87 and 88-97, respectively*). The idea behind these exercises is to remove all tension from the feet or hands, which will, in turn, make the work on the reflex points more beneficial.

After the relaxation exercises, move on to the basic reflexology session. The exercises in the session are designed to make contact with all the major parts and systems of the body – toning and fine tuning their functioning – and so they are an important and integral part of the general health care and maintenance programme central to day-to-day wellbeing. When carrying out the basic session, take note of any reflex points that seem at all sensitive – sensitive reflex points are good indicators of specific health problems. At the end of the session, which should take about 40 to 50 minutes, depending on how experienced you are, go back to the sensitive reflex points you noted and work on these again as described in those chapters. This will probably not extend the session by more than about 5 minutes or so.

In this chapter you will find illustrations of the techniques you need to use for treating specific ailments, such as irritable bowel syndrome, angina, menstrual cramps, back pain, and many others. These are intended to act as a type of shorthand summary and so the detailed description of the precise position of hands, thumbs, fingers, and so on have most often been repeated. If, however, you require more information, then refer to the relevant feet or hand treatment chapters.

Because foot reflexology requires two people – the giver, or practitioner, and the receiver – it is not possible to use it as a self-help therapy, and so the information relating to the feet is of most interest to the reflexology practitioner. However, hand reflexology is a self-help technique and this has also been included to allow you to work on some health problems yourself between foot sessions.

The Digestive System

Because the digestive system has to cope with the great variety of food and drink we ingest, it is very prone to upset and can easily become unbalanced. Stress, too, plays a significant role in the problems associated with the the digestive system (*see pp. 42-5*).

Indigestion
Indigestion is caused by a muscular spasm in the stomach, which, in turn, causes an unbalanced secretion of digestive enzymes. This can result in flatulence and general discomfort, often accompanied by excess acidity.

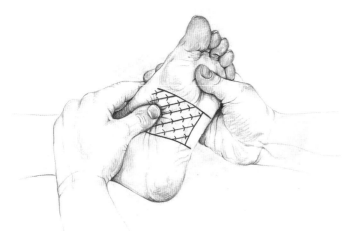

Working the foot
The reflex points to work in order to ease indigestion are the stomach and pancreas. These are found only on the left foot. Support the left foot with your right hand and use your left thumb to work the area indicated.

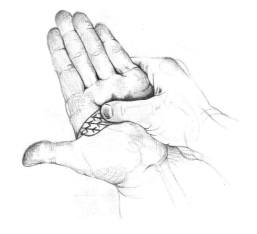

Working the hand
The stomach, pancreas, and spleen reflex points are found only on the left hand. Work on the palm of your left hand with your right thumb in the area indicated, using the usual forward, creeping movement (see p. 36).

Gall stones

Gall stones are small, granular clumps of material that build up in the gallbladder and, if left untreated, can eventually block the bile duct. Bile is secreted into the digestive system to help with the digestion of fat, and it also acts as a lubricant to aid the evacuation of waste products from the bowel. Many people who have undergone gallbladder removal have subsequently suffered from constipation, which had not been a problem in the past. Reflexology can help to eliminate gall stones. Many sufferers have visited reflexologists in order to receive some relief from their condition while waiting for an operation. On being rescreened prior to surgery it was discovered that the stones had dispersed.

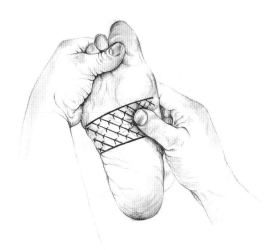

Working the foot
To help ease the pain caused by gall stones, and possibly to assist in their elimination, you need to work the reflex points for the liver and gallbladder, which are found only on the right foot. Supporting the top of the right foot with your left hand, use your right thumb to treat the area indicated.

Working the hand
The reflex points for the liver and gallbladder are found only on your right hand. Rest your right hand on a soft support, such as a comfortable cushion, and use your left thumb to treat the area shown. Work from the lateral to the medial edge.

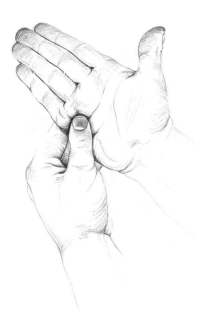

Irritable bowel syndrome

Incidents of irritable bowel syndrome are often accompanied by pain, which can be intense, in the groin or lower abdominal area. This distressing ailment results in some people experiencing constipation, while others have diarrhea. Tension is very often at the seat of these episodes, and many people report a heightening of symptoms prior to an important examination or a job interview. A disturbance in daily routine can also trigger an episode of irritable bowel syndrome, such as switching from day work to night work, or vice versa.

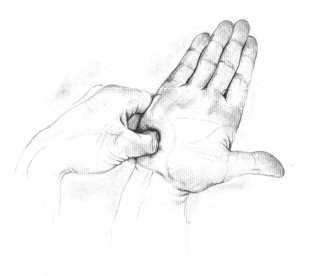

Working the hands

As a first step, use the hooking-out technique (see p. 39) to work out the area of the ileocecal valve (above). Then, commencing with the right hand at the lateral edge of the waist line (right), use the regular thumb technique to work across the palm of the hand in straight lines, right to the heel of the hand. Hand relaxation exercises with greatly enhance the benefit of the treatment.

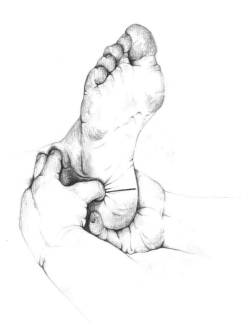

Working the feet
*First, use the hooking-out technique
(see p. 39) on the ileocecal valve (left).*

*Next, starting on the right foot at the
medial edge of the waist line, use your left
thumb to work the area indicated (right)
in straight lines, right to the base of the
heel. Here you will be contacting the reflex
points for the ascending, transverse colon
and small intestines.*

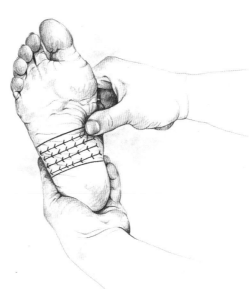

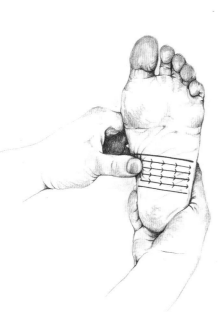

*Changing to the left foot (left), work
in straight lines with your left thumb
from the medial edge of the waist line
right to the base of the heel. This time
you will be contacting the reflex points
for the transverse, descending sigmoid
colon, small intestines, and the rectum.*

The Respiratory System

The main organs of the respiratory system are the two lungs and the connecting air passages from the nose and mouth (*see pp. 50-3*).

Emphysema

This very distressing condition can occur in people who have suffered many years of chronic bronchitis, asthma, and similar lung infections. Emphysema can also occur as a result of working with asbestos and some types of chemical insecticides used in agriculture without using special face masks to protect the lungs.

Emphysema causes a collapse of the tiny air sacs, or alveoli, in the lungs, resulting in a build-up of fluid in the bottom of these organs. This, in turn, restricts the amount of oxygen the lungs can draw in and pass to the bloodstream. As a result, patients can be severely disabled with even the simplest of tasks leaving them gasping for breath. This places the heart under great stress and, apart from using antibiotics to combat the repeated respiratory infections and steroids to break down the inflammation, there is not much that can be done.

The main benefits reflexology can bring to emphysema sufferers lie in easing the stress associated with the condition, increasing lung function as much as possible, and helping to relieve some of the strain on the heart.

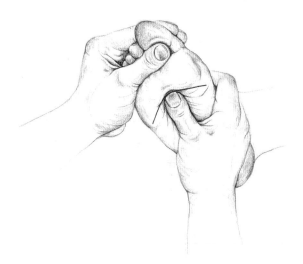

Working the feet

To help lessen the symptoms of emphysema, first start with the basic diaphragm-relaxation exercise. Beginning with the right foot, place your right thumb on the start of the diaphragm line. Move your thumb outward, toward the lateral side of the foot. At the same time, bend the toes downward on to your left thumb. Repeat this exercise for the left foot. This exercise relaxes the large diaphragm muscle situated at the base of the lungs and may ease laboured breathing.

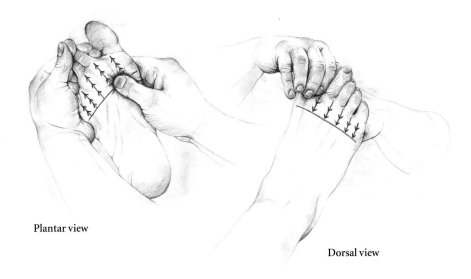

Plantar view

Dorsal view

Next, work on the lung/breast reflex points. On the plantar view (above), support the right foot with your left hand, and work up the area from the base of the diaphragm line to where the toes join the foot. On the dorsal view (above right), make a fist with your left hand and press it into the plantar side side of the right foot, and use your right index finger to work down the foot in the grooves. Repeat these steps on the left foot.

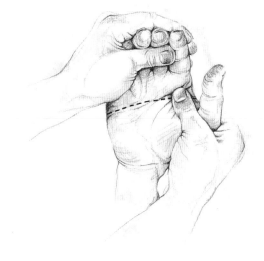

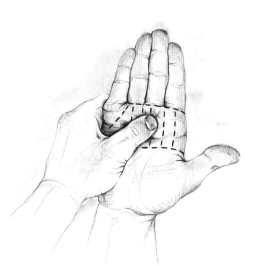

Working the hands

For the diaphragm-relaxation exercise (above) you will need the help of an assistant, but it is excellent for relaxing the respiratory system (see p. 90). To work the lung reflex points (left), place your left thumb on the diaphragm line of your right hand. Work up in straight lines to where the fingers join the hand. Repeat for the left hand.

The Heart

Central to the circulatory system is the heart. This organ ensures that every cell in the body is served with an oxygen-enriched blood supply (*see pp. 54-5*).

Angina

Angina is thought to result from lack of exercise, a high-fat diet, and stress. However, hereditary factors may also be involved. The disease itself causes corrosion of the walls of the arteries, leading to a build-up of pressure and severe chest pains as the blood tries to flow through the restricted openings.

Working the feet and hand

The heart reflex is found only on the left foot (left). Supporting the left foot with your right hand, use your left thumb to work the area in horizontal lines. The rib-cage relaxation exercise (below– see also p. 79) is also very beneficial. To treat angina as a self-help technique, rest your left hand on a pillow and work over the area of the heart reflex points with your right thumb (below left).

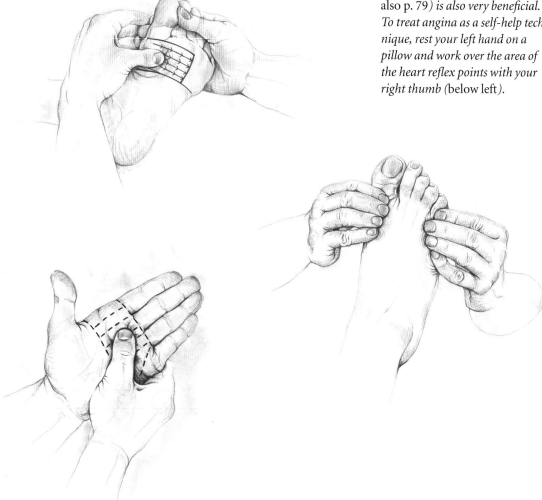

Palpitations

Palpitations, or a racing heart, are not uncommon. Sometimes they can be a symptom of a heart condition so always consult your doctor if you are at all concerned. Other causes of palpitations include food allergies and excess caffeine or alcohol, but very often palpitations are brought on through anxiety and stress.

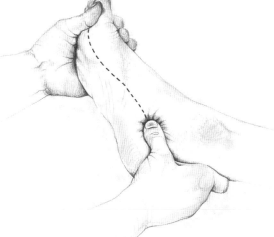

Working the feet

First, run through all of the relaxation exercises to help de-stress the receiver (see pp. 77-9). Next, it helps to work the spine, which is a link to the central nervous system (left). Supporting the right foot with your left hand, work up the spinal reflex points and into the brain, using your right thumb. Repeat for the left foot. To treat the heart reflex point, see opposite.

Working the hands

For the spine reflex points on your right hand (below left), work along the line indicated with your left thumb. Repeat for your left hand. To work the right side of the brain (below), apply pressure with your left thumb to the top of your right thumb. Repeat for your left hand.

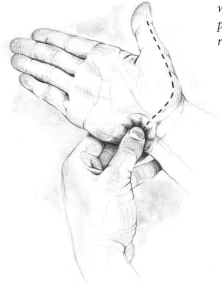

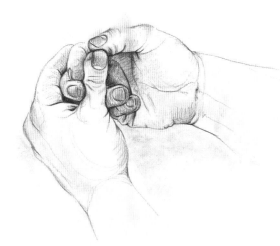

The Lymphatic System

One of the main functions of the body's lymphatic system is to filter out bacteria and other harmful substances. This process can lead to inflammation of the lymph nodes (*see pp. 56-7*).

Fluid retention

Many women suffer from fluid retention at certain stages of their menstrual cycle each month, resulting in puffiness of the fingers and ankles, for example, and a general feeling of being "bloated".

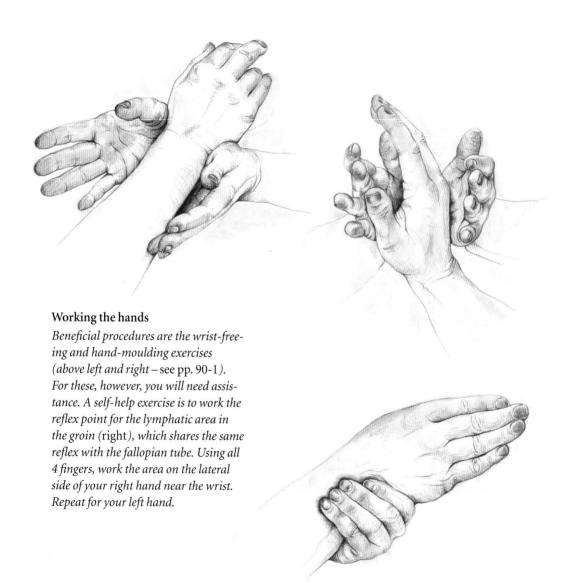

Working the hands

Beneficial procedures are the wrist-freeing and hand-moulding exercises (above left and right – see pp. 90-1). For these, however, you will need assistance. A self-help exercise is to work the reflex point for the lymphatic area in the groin (right), which shares the same reflex with the fallopian tube. Using all 4 fingers, work the area on the lateral side of your right hand near the wrist. Repeat for your left hand.

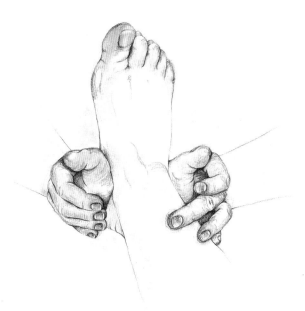

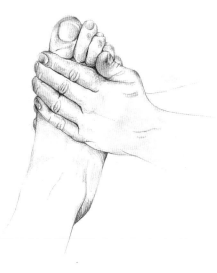

Working the feet

Swollen or painful feet can be relieved by using the ankle-freeing (top) and foot-moulding (right) warm-up exercises (see pp. 77 and 79).

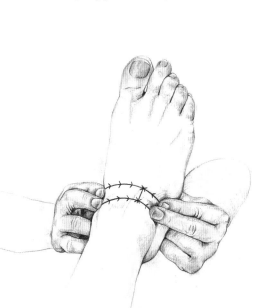

Next, work the lymphatic area (left), which shares its reflex points with the fallopian tube. This is a beneficial area to treat to relieve tight discomfort in the feet. Starting on the right foot, press into the soles of the foot with both of your thumbs and work over the front of the foot with the index fingers of both of your hands. Repeat this technique on the left foot.

The Endocrine System

Many of the glands making up the endocrine system are extremely susceptible to being thrown out of balance by physiological or emotional stresses on the body (*see pp. 58-61*).

Menstrual cramps and thyroid disorders

Although menstrual cramps can be a factor in the life of any pre-menopausal woman, young teenagers are particular sufferers. The activity of the thyroid gland – and thus the production of the hormone, thyroxine – is under the control of the particular hormone manufactured by the pituitary. Any imbalance in the amount of thyroxine can lead to dramatic changes in metabolism and behaviour.

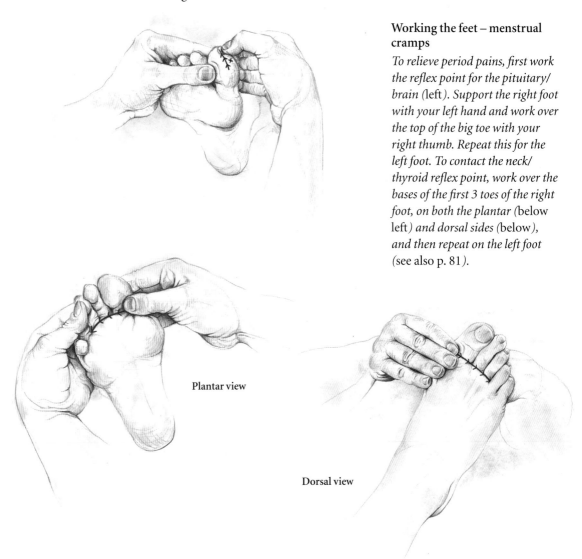

Working the feet – menstrual cramps

To relieve period pains, first work the reflex point for the pituitary/ brain (left). Support the right foot with your left hand and work over the top of the big toe with your right thumb. Repeat this for the left foot. To contact the neck/ thyroid reflex point, work over the bases of the first 3 toes of the right foot, on both the plantar (below left) and dorsal sides (below), and then repeat on the left foot (see also p. 81).

Plantar view

Dorsal view

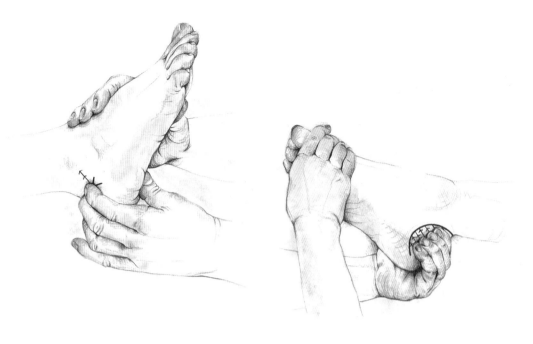

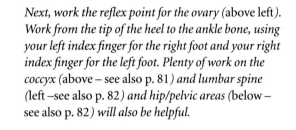

Next, work the reflex point for the ovary (above left).
Work from the tip of the heel to the ankle bone, using
your left index finger for the right foot and your right
index finger for the left foot. Plenty of work on the
coccyx (above – see also p. 81) and lumbar spine
(left –see also p. 82) and hip/pelvic areas (below –
see also p. 82) will also be helpful.

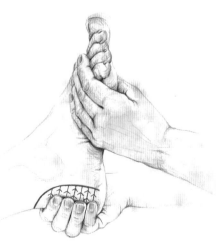

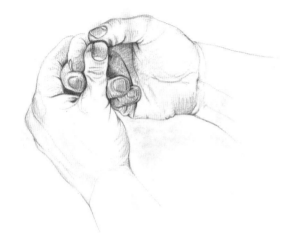

Working the hands – menstrual cramps

As a self-help therapy for menstrual cramp, or period pain, first work the reflex point for the brain/pituitary area (left). For the right side of the brain, apply pressure directly to the top of your right thumb with your left thumb. Repeat this on your left hand to work the left side of the brain.

The next helpful exercise is to work the reflex points in the area of the ovaries (right). Work over the area on the lateral side of your right hand (just in front of the wrist bone) with the second finger of your left hand. Repeat this for your left hand, using the second finger of your right hand to work the reflex points.

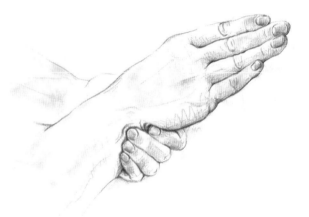

114

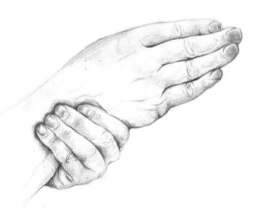

To contact the reflex points for the fallopian tube (left), use pressure from all 4 fingers of your left hand, work over the area on the lateral side of your right hand. Repeat this procedure for your left hand.

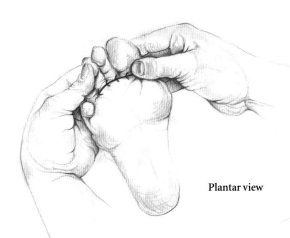

Plantar view

Working the feet – thyroid disorders

To help to normalize the functioning of the thyroid, work on the bases of the first 3 toes on each foot. First, work on the plantar side of the right foot (left), using your right thumb, Then work the left foot, using your left thumb. On the dorsal side of each foot (below), use your index finger to work the area where the toes join the foot.

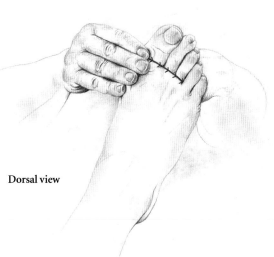

Dorsal view

Plantar view

Working the hands – thyroid disorders

To treat the plantar side of the neck/ thyroid reflex point in the hand (above), use your left thumb just at the bases of the first 3 fingers on your right hand. On the dorsal side (right), use your thumb to work the area where the fingers join the hand.

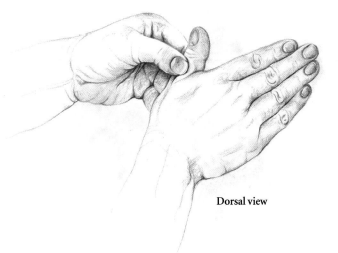

Dorsal view

The Central Nervous System

This system is like a telephone network, with the brain as the exchange sending information to every part of the body along nerves channelled through the spinal cord (*see pp. 68-71*).

Multiple sclerosis

Although at present an incurable degenerative condition of the central nervous system, some of the discomfort associated with multiple sclerosis can be eased by reflexology. Muscular spasms can sometimes be lessened in frequency and severity, for example, and the distressing weakness in the entire body can often be improved.

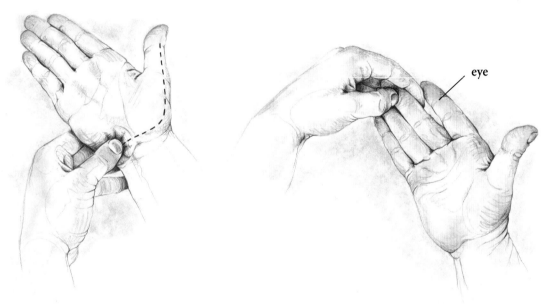

eye

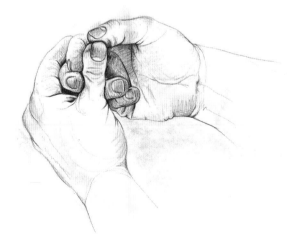

Working the hands

To work the spinal region reflex points (above), start on the lateral side of your right hand and use your thumb to work along the entire line indicated, right to the top of the thumb. For the eye and ear reflex points (above right), start on your right hand and use the rotating technique (see p. 39) on your second and third fingers. To treat the facial areas (right), use your left index finger to work down from the fingernail of your right thumb to the first joint. Repeat all of these for your left hand.

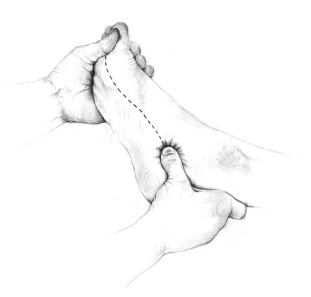

Working the feet

To treat the spinal regions on the foot (left), support the top of the right foot with your left hand, and use your left thumb to work up the reflex points corresponding to the spinal vertebrae on the medial side. Repeat this for the left foot.

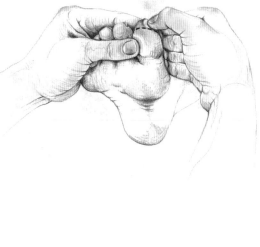

For the brain area (right), support the right foot with left hand and work over the top of the big toe with your right thumb. Repeat this for the left foot, using your left thumb to work the reflex points.

ear

To work the eye and ear reflex points (left), use a rotating action of your thumb (see p. 39) on the reflex points on the second and third toes. Repeat this procedure for the left foot.

The Skeletal System

Reflexology has been successful in relaxing muscles and inflammation in nerve pathways resulting from imbalances in the skeletal system and in normalizing the working of the spine (*see pp. 62-7*).

Back pain
It is pain in the back that motivates most people to seek help from reflexology. If the pain is related to the right side of the spine, expect the reflex points on the right side of the foot or hand to be sensitive; if the pain is on the left of the spine, then the sensitivity will be restricted to the reflex points on the left foot or hand.

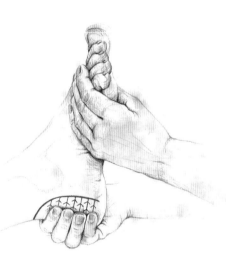

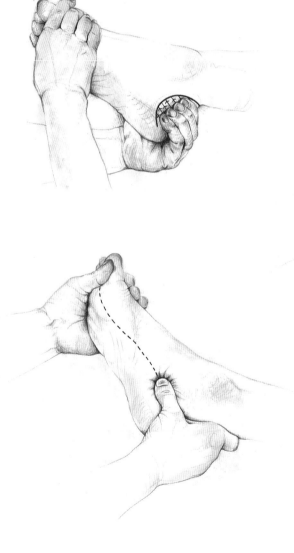

Working the feet
For the coccyx (above left), use all 4 fingers on the medial side of the right foot. Repeat for the left foot. To treat the hip and pelvic areas (above), work on the lateral side of each foot with all 4 fingers, starting on the right foot. For the spinal area (left), support the top of the right foot with your left hand, and use your right thumb to work up the reflex points corresponding to the spinal vertebrae on the medial side.

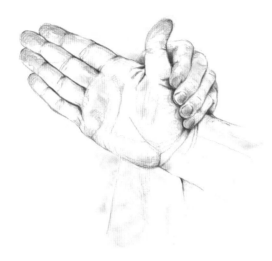

Working the hands

Starting at the medial edge of the plantar side of your hand, work the reflex point corresponding to the coccyx (above– see also p. 93), and then move on to hip and pelvic reflex points (right – see also p. 93).

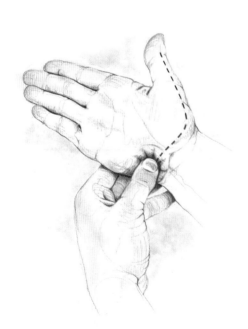

For the spinal reflex points (left – see also p. 94), work the area indicated with your thumb. Use exactly the same techniques when working your left hand.

The joints

The body has a variety of joints – a saddle joint, for example, allows movement in two directions without rotation, hinge joints allow extension and flexion, while ball-and-socket joints move freely in all directions. Because of the constant wear on the joints caused by movement and, in some cases, weight bearing, the joints are susceptible to many painful complaints. Two common problem areas are the hip joint and the shoulder.

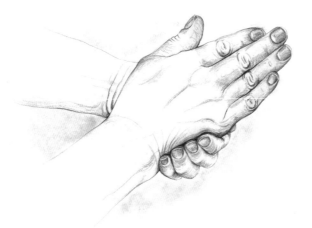

The hip joint

The reflex points for the hip and pelvic region are on the dorsal side of the hand on the lateral edge (above). Use all 4 fingers to work this part of your hand and then repeat for your left hand. To work the feet (right), start with the right foot and use all 4 fingers to work the area indicated. Repeat this technique for the left foot.

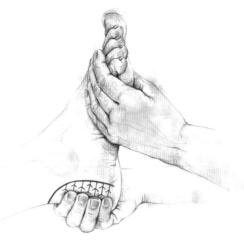

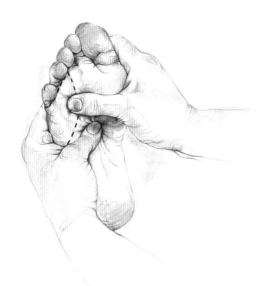

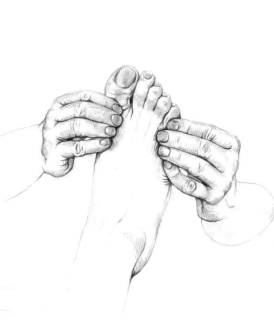

Frozen shoulder

The shoulder reflex points are on the lateral edge of the foot, just under the area of the fifth toe (above) and in the same position on the hand (above right). Work this area on each foot or hand. Relaxing the rib cage may also help (right and below). Starting on the right foot or hand, press in with both thumbs and use all the fingers of both of your hands to creep around to the dorsal side. Start on the right hand or foot and repeat on the left.

The Urinary System

The function of the urinary system is to filter waste products and impurities from the body before they can build up to toxic levels. Apart from the kidneys, the other main parts of the urinary system are the ureter tubes and and bladder (*see pp. 74-5*).

Cystitis

Mainly affecting women, cystitis is an inflammatory condition of the bladder. It causes low pelvic pain and discomfort, frequent urination, and feelings of being generally unwell.

Working the feet

*The first step is to work the bladder reflex point (*left*), using your right thumb on the puffy area on the medial edge of the foot. Repeat for the left foot. To treat the ureter (*below*), locate its reflex point on the medial side of the ligament line. Be careful to avoid applying pressure on the ligament line itself. Repeat for the left foot. Finally, apply thumb pressure directly to the kidney reflex point (*below left*) and then rotate the foot around it. Repeat for the left foot.*

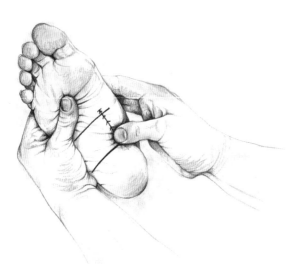

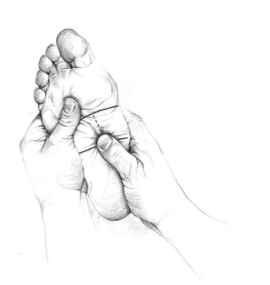

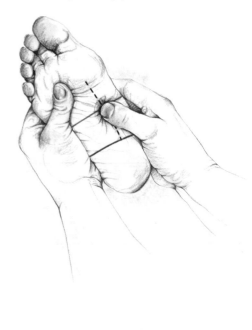

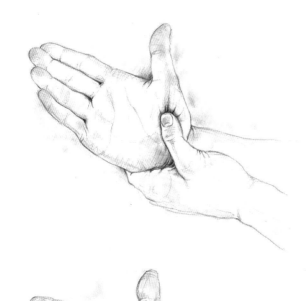

Working the hands

To contact the bladder reflex point (left), apply thumb pressure to the fleshy pad below the thumb. Repeat for the left hand. For the ureter (below left), still using your thumb, continue from the bladder reflex point toward the base of the index finger, and repeat for the left hand. Finally, you will find the kidney reflex point (below) where the thumb joins the hand. Repeat for the left hand.

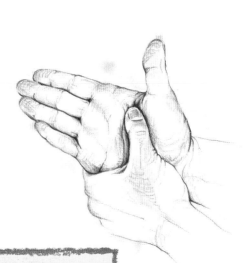

Renal colic

Renal, or kidney, colic is caused by small particles of sand-like material that accumulate in the kidneys. This condition can lead to the formation of kidney stones. The pain associated with renal colic is often extremely severe and may need to be treated with injections of such painkillers as morphine. Temporary relief can be found by flushing your system through with large quantities of fluids taken by mouth but, unfortunately, renal colic tends to recur. Reflexology has proved to be very effective in giving long-term relief from the pain associated with this condition, and the reflex points you should target are the same as those for cystitis. These reflex points stimulate your entire urinary system, increasing its efficiency.

Psychosomatic Ailments

Many people think the term "psychosomatic" refers to imaginary, and therefore "not real", ailments; here, however, it describes those disorders that are either brought on by, or are aggravated by, stress.

Premenstrual tension

Symptoms ranging from feelings of being "out of sorts" to depression and violent mood swings can accompany premenstrual tension, while physical ailments include painful and swollen breasts, fluid retention, and tiredness. The benefits of reflexology lie in its ability to correct hormonal imbalances, relax the body and spirit, and help with the elimination of excess fluid from the body.

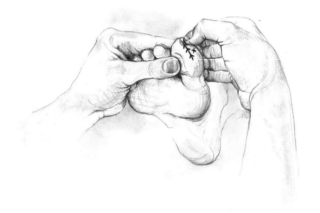

Working the feet

Premenstrual tension can be helped by targeting the endocrine and reproductive systems and, specifically, by working the reflex points for the neck/thyroid (see p. 81), the brain (above – see also p. 82), and the ovaries (right – see also p. 87).

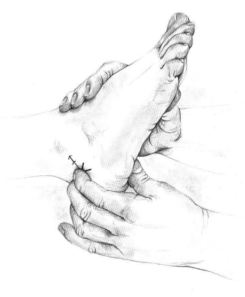

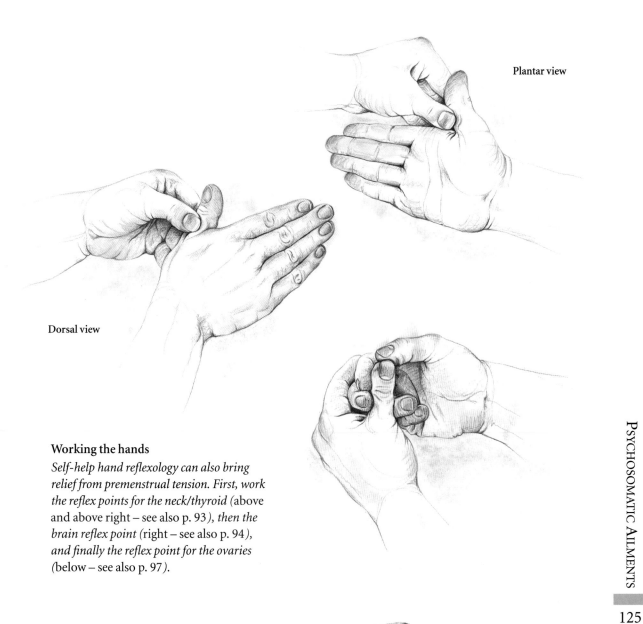

Plantar view

Dorsal view

Working the hands

Self-help hand reflexology can also bring relief from premenstrual tension. First, work the reflex points for the neck/thyroid (above and above right – see also p. 93), then the brain reflex point (right – see also p. 94), and finally the reflex point for the ovaries (below – see also p. 97).

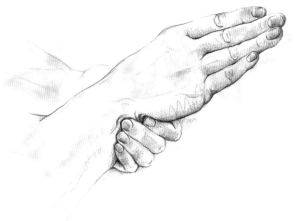

Depression

Weekly sessions of reflexology over a period of about three months can work wonders for those suffering from depression. This illness often centres around suppressed anger, and if sufferers cannot deal with it they may retreat into a protective shell to avoid the disturbing feeling and emotions that are aroused. Working the respiratory and circulatory systems has a great calming effect, and the use of all the relaxation techniques will also be beneficial in bringing about a general feeling of wellbeing.

Working the feet

The most direct way of treating the respiratory system is to contact the reflex points for the lung/breast area (far left and left). On the plantar side, work up from the base of the diaphragm line to the join of the toes to the foot. On the dorsal side, make a fist and press it into the sole and use your index finger to work down the groove.

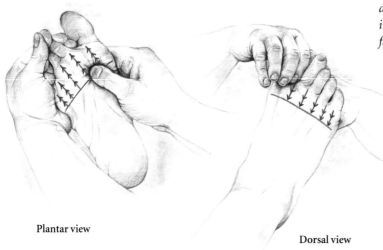

Plantar view

Dorsal view

For the circulatory system (right), you will find the heart reflex point in the area shown, but only on the left foot. Support the top of the foot with your right hand and use your left thumb to work the area from the medial edge. Follow on from this with some diaphragm-relaxation exercises (see p. 77).

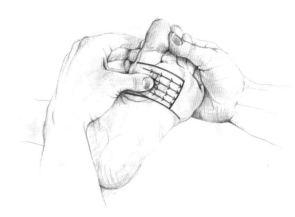

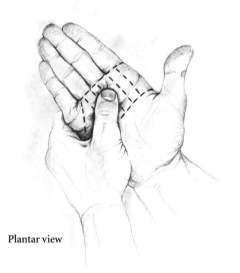

Plantar view

Working the hands

As a self-help therapy for depression, first contact the reflex points for the lungs. On the plantar side (left), start on your right hand and use your left thumb to work in straight lines from the diaphragm line to where your fingers join your hand. Repeat on the left hand.

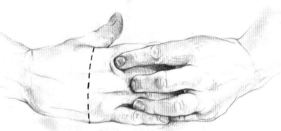

Dorsal view

On the dorsal side (right), place your left index finger at the join of your fingers to your right hand, and work down the hand for about 1½in (4cm). Repeat on your left hand.

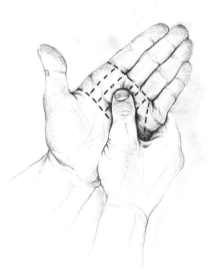

For the heart reflex point (left), which is found only on your left hand, work the area indicated with your right thumb. If you have a helper, follow this with some diaphragm-relaxation exercises (see p. 90).

Allergies

Allergic reactive conditions are often linked to stress. The more tension and anxiety we experience, the less efficiently our bodies cope with the scores of potential irritants in the food we eat, the water we drink, and the air we breathe. If, however, you discover that your allergic reaction is very specific – say, to a certain type of food – the best course of action is to avoid the allergen whenever possible.

The benefits of treating allergic conditions with reflexology lie in its ability to toughen up the digestive system to cope with irritants and to relax the nervous system so that it is more efficient.

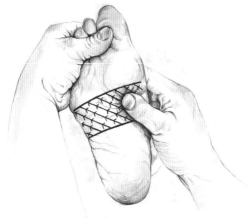

128

Working the feet

The reflex points for the liver (above) are found only on the right foot. While supporting the right foot with your left hand, use your right thumb to work the area indicated. The reflex point for the ileocecal valve (right) is, again, only on the right foot. Supporting the right foot by the heel with your right hand, use the hooking-out technique (see p. 39) with your left thumb.

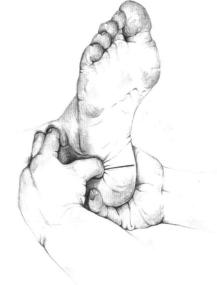

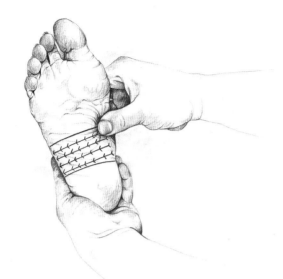

To work the transverse and ascending colon and small intestines (left), support the right foot with your left hand and use your right thumb to work across the foot in straight lines right to the base of the heel.

For the stomach and pancreas reflex points (right), work on the left foot only. While supporting the left foot with your right hand, use your left thumb to work the area indicated.

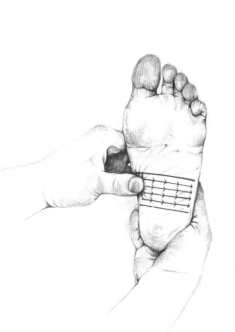

Finally, for the transverse and descending colon (left), treat the left foot, supporting it with your right hand, and using your left thumb to work across the foot to the base of the heel.

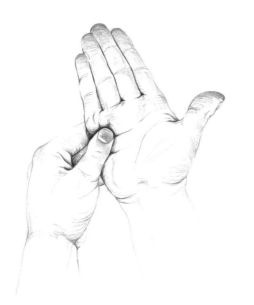

Working the hands

The type of self-help procedures suitable for combating allergic reactions basically mirror those for the feet (see pp. 128-9). To work the reflex points representing the liver (left), rest your right hand comfortably on a supporting surface, such as a cushion, and use your left thumb to work over the area indicated. This helps generally to detoxify the body and greatly assists in curbing allergic reactions, such as hay fever and skin reactions.

In order to stimulate both the small and large intestines, use the hooking-out technique (see p. 39) on the reflex point for the ileocecal valve (right). This point is found on your right hand and is worked using your left thumb. As with the liver exercise, this also helps the body eliminate waste products.

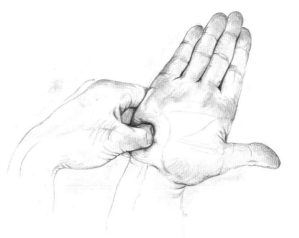

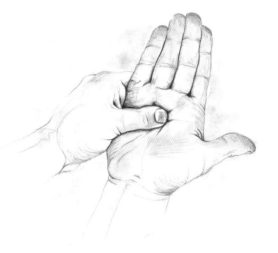

To work the transverse and ascending colon (left), work across the palm of your right hand in the area indicated, following the direction of the arrows.

For the reflex points governing the stomach, pancreas, and spleen (right), you must work on your left hand only. Using the thumb of your right hand, work out the area indicated on your left palm.

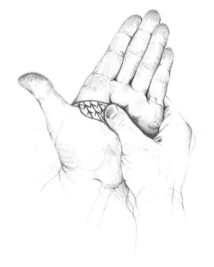

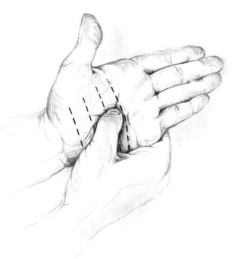

Finally, for the transverse and descending colon (left), work on the palm of your left hand using your right thumb as indicated.

Arthritis

Arthritis is not a single disease but a group of conditions commonly classified as being either rheumatoid arthritis, which affects the musculo-skeletal system, or osteo-arthritis, a chronic disease of the joints. Arthritis in one form or another, and to one degree or another, affects 75 per cent of people over the age of 50.

This condition is not new. In Ancient Rome, arthritis was considered to be such a burden that the Emperor Diocletian exempted citizens suffering with severe arthritis from paying taxes.

Use reflexology to treat those parts of the skeletal system (*see pp. 62-7 and the relevant Treatment chapters*) that are affected – mainly the knees, neck, hands, hips, and spine, plus the digestive system.

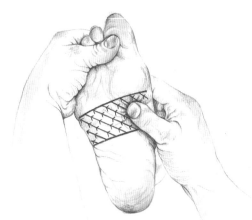

Working the feet
To contact the reflex points for the liver (left), *support the right foot with your left hand and work the area indicated in the direction of the arrows.*

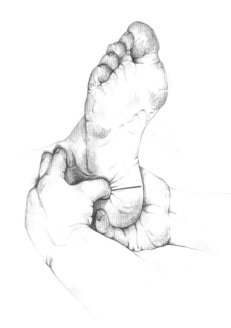

The reflex point for the ileocecal valve (right) *is only on the right foot. Supporting the right foot by the heel with your right hand, use the hooking-out technique (see p. 39) with your left thumb.*

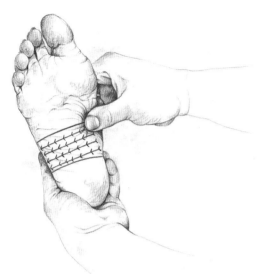

To work the transverse and ascending colon and small intestines (left), support the right foot with your left hand and use your right thumb to work across the foot in straight lines right to the base of the heel.

For the stomach and pancreas reflex points (right), work on the left foot only. While supporting the left foot with your right hand, use your left thumb to work the area indicated.

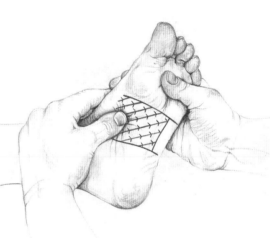

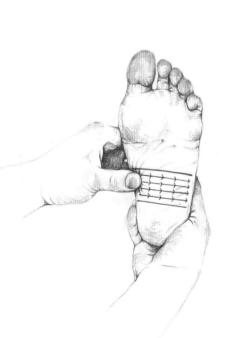

Finally, for the transverse and descending colon (left), work on the left foot, supporting it with your right hand, and using your left thumb to work across the foot to the base of the heel.

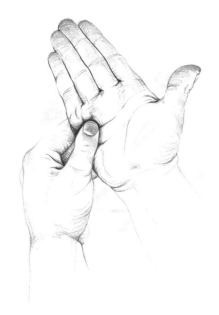

Working the hands

The types of self-help procedures suitable for combating arthritis concentrate on stimulating the body's ability to eliminate waste products. To work the reflex points representing the liver (left), rest your right hand comfortably on a supporting surface, such as a cushion, and use your left thumb to work over the area indicated. This helps generally to detoxify the body.

In order to stimulate both the small and large intestines, use the hooking-out technique (see p. 39) on the reflex point for the ileocecal valve (right). This point is found on your right hand and is worked using your left thumb. As with the liver exercise, this also helps the body eliminate waste products.

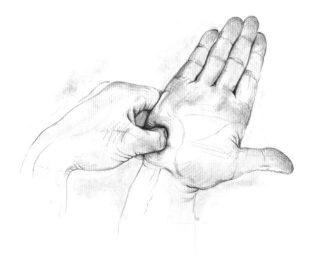

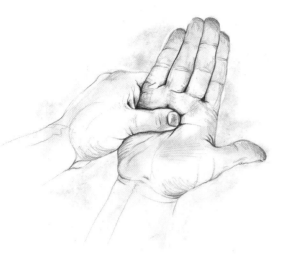

To work the transverse and ascending colon (left), work across the palm of your right hand in the area indicated, following the direction of the arrows.

For the reflex points governing the stomach, pancreas, and spleen (right), you must work on the left hand only. Using the thumb of your right hand, work out the area indicated on your left palm.

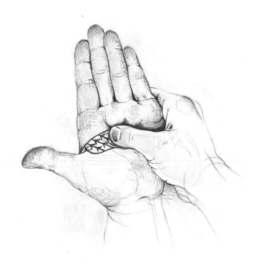

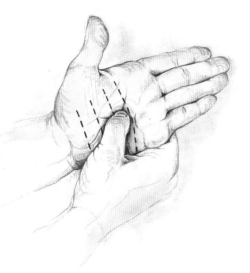

Finally, for the transverse and descending colon (left), work on the palm of your left hand using your right thumb as indicated.

Ailments Reference Chart

CONDITION	SYMPTOMS	MAIN AREAS TO TREAT
Alzheimer's disease	Degeneration of the cerebral cortex, leading to loss of memory and paralysis	Extensive work on all of spine and brain, preferably daily
Angina	Chest/heart pain often radiating down the arm and up to the face	Respiratory and circulatory systems
Ankylosing spondylitis	Disease of the joints, destruction of joint space followed by sclerosis and calcification, resulting in rigidity of spinal column and thorax	Spine, brain, shoulder, hip, knee, coccyx and pelvis – also adrenals to help break down the inflammation
Arthritis	Pain and swelling in joints	Area of pain, plus digestive and endocrine systems
Bronchitis and asthma	Inflammation of bronchial tubes, and spasm of the bronchioles resulting in difficulty in exhalation	Heart/lung, adrenals, thoracic spine (to help nerve supply to this area), digestive system (a weakness in the digestive system may cause excessive mucus)
Bursitis and gout	Inflammation of the bursa of a joint	Work the relevant joint – i.e. the knee or elbow – plus lumbar spine for the knee or cervical spine for the elbow (to help the nerve supply to the affected part)
Candida	A fungus that causes thrush	The whole of the intestinal area and reproductive system
Carcinoma (cancer)	Cancer of the epithelial tissue	The whole of the body, but especially the spleen (to help the immune system)
Carpal tunnel syndrome	Numbness and tingling in the fingers and hand as the result of compression of the median nerve of the wrist	Cervical spine and elbow area (to aid nerve supply to wrist)
Cataract	Opacity of the lens of the eye	Eye, sinuses, and cervical spine
Cerebral hemorrhage (stroke)	Rupture of an artery of the brain due to either high blood pressure or disease of the artery	Entire spine, brain, respiratory and circulatory systems and kidneys (to help the renal blood supply and so ultimately help to reduce blood pressure)
Cerebral palsy (spasticity)	Condition in which the control of the motor system is affected due to a lesion resulting from a birth defect or deprivation of oxygen at birth	The spine and brain (work this area frequently during treatment – 6 or 7 times up and down each foot)

Cervical spondylosis	Degenerative changes in the inter-vertebral discs in the cervical spine	The entire spine and neck area
Colitis, diverticulitis, and irritable bowel syndrome	Inflammation of the colon	Entire digestive system and lumbar spine (to help nerve and blood supply to the pelvic area)
Conjunctivitis (eye condition)	Inflammation of the conjunctiva	Eye/cervical spine and all sinus areas
Constipation	Difficulty in passing a motion	Entire intestine and liver/gallbladder areas (bile helps lubrication of the bowel) and lumbar spinal nerves
Crohn's disease	Chronic form of enteritis affecting ter-minal part of the ileum	Entire intestinal area
Cystitis	Inflammation of the urinary system, mainly affecting the bladder	Urinary system, as well as the coccyx, pelvis, and lumbar spine
Depression	A feeling of gloom, despondency, and apathy	Entire endocrine system, to help balance hormonal output, and lots of work on relaxation techniques
Diabetes	Caused by a deficiency of insulin pro-duction of the pancreas.	Digestive, endocrine, circulatory, and respiratory systems
Dysmenorrhea	Painful or difficult menstruation	Urinary and reproductive systems and coccyx/pelvis and lumbar spine
Eczema and all skin diseases	Inflammation of the skin	Treat as for asthma (they stem from the same problem)
Edema	Abnormal amount of fluid in the tissues causing swelling, particularly in ankles	Urinary and circulatory systems, lumbar spine, and lymphatic area surrounding the groin
Emphysema	The over-distension of the lungs by air. Distension of the alveoli of the lungs due to atrophy of the alveolar walls.	Treat as for asthma
Endometriosis	Inflammation of the endometrium (uterus)	Reproductive and endocrine systems (can result from a hormone imbalance)
Epilepsy	Disorder of the brain marked by the occurrence of convulsive fits	Brain and entire spine
Fibroid	A tumour composed of mixed muscular and fibrous tissue in the uterus	Reproductive system

CONDITION	SYMPTOMS	MAIN AREAS TO TREAT
Glandular fever	Infectious illness of the glandular system	Endocrine, respiratory, and circulatory systems
Hay fever	Inflammation of the mucus membrane lining of the nose	Sinus, ear, eye, and adrenals
Headache	Pain in head	Entire spine and brain
Hemorrhoids	Varicose veins in the rectum	Intestinal area, in particular the descending colon and rectum
Hypertension	High blood pressure	Circulatory and respiratory systems and kidneys. **Do not** work on the adrenals when treating high blood pressure
Hypotension	Low blood pressure	As above, but work on the adrenals to increase blood pressure
Incontinence	Absence of voluntary control of the passing of urine or faeces	Urinary/intestinal, lumbar spine, coccyx, and pelvis
Indigestion	Failure of the digestive process	Digestive system and intestinal areas
Insomnia	Inability to sleep	Spine, brain, and respiratory and circulatory systems
Lumbago	Painful condition of the lumbar muscles due to inflammation	Coccyx, pelvis, lumbar spine (may be caused by displaced intervertebral disc)
Mastitis	Inflammation of the breast	Breast, shoulder, and endocrine system
Meniere's disease	Giddiness resulting from a disease of the inner ear	Head, sinuses, ear, cervical spine, and neck
Migraine	Sudden, recurring attacks of headache, usually with nausea, preceded by disorders of vision	Head, neck, spine, and liver (migraine is often digestive in origin and so the liver is usually affected)
Multiple sclerosis	Degeneration of the myelin sheath covering central nervous system	Spine and brain
Nephritis	Inflammation of the kidney	Urinary system and lumbar spine
Neuralgia	Pain in the nerves of the face	Facial area, cervical spine, and all sinuses

Osteo-arthritis	Disorder due to excessive wear and tear of joint surfaces, affecting mainly the weight-bearing joints	Work thoroughly the prime joint or part of the body affected, as well as the spine and urinary system (to encourage good elimination)
Pancreatitis	Inflammation of the pancreas	Digestive system
Phlebitis	Inflammation of the veins	Circulatory and respiratory systems
Prostatitis	Prostate inflammation	Urinary and reproductive systems, also the lumbar spine
Retinitis	Inflammation of the retina	Eye, sinuses, and neck
Rhinitis, or hay fever	Inflammation of mucus lining of the nose	Sinuses, nose/throat, digestive system (often a food allergy), and adrenals (to reduce inflammation)
Salpingitis	Inflammation of the fallopian tubes	Entire reproductive and endocrine systems, plus the coccyx, pelvic/hip
Sciatica	Neuralgia of the sciatic nerve	Lumbar spine, coccyx, pelvic/hip, and sciatic area
Sinusitis	Inflammation of an air sinus	Sinuses, eye/ear, cervical spine, facial area
Spondylitis (as in ankylosing spondylitis)	Inflammation of a vertebra – the condition occurs characteristically in young men, leading to ossification of the spinal ligaments with ankylosis of the cervical and sacro-iliac joints	Entire skeletal system
Tennis elbow	Inflammation of the bursa of a joint, affecting the insertion of the extensor tendon of the forearm muscles	Cervical spine, shoulder, and elbow
Thrombosis	Coagulation of blood in the vessels	Respiratory and circulatory systems, plus spine
Tinnitus	Ringing in the ears	Neck, ear, and sinuses
Tonsillitis	Inflammation of the tonsils	Throat, sinuses, cervical spine (to help immunity in young children
Trigeminal neuralgia	Pains in the face – of unknown cause	Face, sinuses, eye/ear, and neck
Vertigo	Giddiness	Ear, sinuses, and cervical spine

Index

Useful addresses & further reading

If you would like to know more about reflexology or consult a reflexologist, contact any of the following organizations:

International Institute of Reflexology, PO Box 12642, St Petersburg, Florida, FLA 33733-2642
American Reflexology Certification Board (ARCB), POBox 620607, Littleton, CO 80162 (303-933-6921)
International Council of Reflexologists (ICR), C/O 4400 El Parque Ave., Las Vegas, NV 89102
Ohio Association of Reflexologists (OAR), POBox 428725, Cincinnati, OH 45242
Pennsylvania Reflexology Association (PRA), 1900 Emerson Street, Philadelphia, PA 19152
Reflexology Association of California (RAC), POBox 641156, Los Angeles, CA 90064
Associated Reflexologists of Colorado (ARC), POBox 471812, Aurora, CO 80047
Maine Council of Reflexologists (MCR), POBox 969, Jefferson, ME 04348
Missouri State Reflexology Association (MSRA), 12817 East 47th, 17 Grove, Independence, MO 64055

Further Reading
Byers, Dwight C., Better Health with Foot Reflexology (Ingham Publishing 1983)
Ingham, Eunice D., Stories the Feet Can Tell (Ingham Publishing 1938); Stories the Feet Have Told (Ingham Publishing 1951)
Norman, Laura, Feet First: A Guide to Foot Reflexology (Simon & Schuster 1988)

Gaia Books Limited

Books from Gaia celebrate the vision of Gaia, the self-sustaining living Earth, and seek to help its readers live in greater personal and planetary harmony.

Welcome to Gaia – the publisher that leads the world in books on natural health, care of mind, body and spirit, and personal and planetary ecology. Gaia books not only inspire and delight on all these themes but they also inform, entertain, and become bestsellers! They are fun, beautiful, and much loved. Excellence, with that enticing bit of difference, is the Gaia hallmark.

The company took its name from Gaia, the Greek goddess of the Earth, and has been inspired by the Gaia theory developed by scientists James Lovelock and Lynn Margulis in the 1970s and 1980s. This theory proposes that the biosphere, made up of living things, rocks, water, and air, is a kind living organism which can regulate its temperature, atmospheric gas composition, and fluid chemistry. This organism, called Gaia, is powered by the Sun and profoundly influenced by the Moon. She is able to recover from severe damage and can recycle her wastes. While the Gaia theory has faced stiff opposition from some establishment quarters, no one has any doubt that it has encouraged a radical rethinking of the way we view our planetary home.

In more than 12 years of co-edition publishing, Gaia Books has established an extraordinary and unique track record for commercial success combined with integrity of vision. We have brought holistic healing from the fringes to centre stage with our books on massage, yoga, aromatherapy, homeopathy, herbalism and Tai Chi. We have blended health and environment in elegant books, such as *The Natural House Book*, for the new consumer. And we have pioneered answers to global questions with groundbreaking titles such as *The Gaia Atlas of Planet Management*. The high regard in which our books are held is demonstrated by our collaboration with major international organizations, such as UNESCO and OXFAM.

As the millennium approaches, Gaia is again leading the way, helping to bring fresh concerns on to the agenda. We address new spiritual needs and stress that the reawakening of forgotten skills and wisdom is essential to our happiness and survival.